the LANGUAGE
of FRACTURES

the LANGUAGE

of FRACTURES

Robert Jordan Schultz, M.D., F.A.C.S.

Director of Orthopaedic Surgery
Hospital of the Albert Einstein College of Medicine

Associate Professor of Orthopaedic Surgery
Albert Einstein College of Medicine
Bronx, New York

ROBERT E. KRIEGER PUBLISHING CO.
MALABAR, FLORIDA

Original edition 1972
Reprint 1976, 1979, 1983

Printed and Published by
ROBERT E. KRIEGER PUBLISHING CO., INC.
KRIEGER DRIVE
MALABAR, FLA   32950

Printed in the United States of America

Library of Congress Cataloging in Publication Data

Schultz, Robert Jordan.
    The language of fractures.

    Reprint of the ed. published by Williams and Wil-
kins, Baltimore.
    Bibliography: p.
    Includes index.
    1. Fractures. 2. Fractures--Terminology.
I. Title.
RD101.S39 1976   617'.15   75-43698
ISBN 0-88275-369-X

Dedicated to my wife Marcie,
daughter Judy, and my parents
Dr. and Mrs. Abraham Schultz.

FOREWORD

This is a book on fractures with a unique and different approach. First, it introduces a vocabulary concerning fractures and then gives instructions as to how to apply this vocabulary to specific regions. The third portion of the book deals with "Fracture Eponyms," and the final portion concerns itself with "Fractures That Are Not Fractures."

At first this somewhat unorthodox approach seemed a bit unusual, but as I read the manuscript I realized how well the author has not only introduced the principles of diagnosis and treatment of fractures, but subtly established a solid foundation in anatomy and pathology on which these principles are based.

The author's primary goal is to make it possible for the medical student, and hence the physician, to be able at least to describe a fracture accurately. I am not certain whether such skills, once acquired, will succeed in "securing prompt and proper management of fractures" and expedite care in the emergency room; however, I am certain that this book should go a long way toward improving communications, which is always the weakest link in any endeavor.

This book is directed to the undergraduate student, but even the most experienced fracture surgeon will find this "bibliography of eponyms" an interesting and welcome reference from which he can learn a great deal. I believe that this should fill a gap that exists in modern undergraduate medical education with its core curriculum, in which the medical students are learning less and less about more and more, to the point that they soon will know nothing about everything. At least this book should make it possible for the student to convey what he has learned more accurately.

JACK WICKSTROM, M.D.

PREFACE

In this exceedingly hurried world, our endeavors to condense and include tremendous amounts of material into medical school curricula are beset by many difficulties. With the medical school course limited to four years, and a tremendous amount of didactic material to cover, in certain areas, particularly the surgical specialties, only the surface can be scratched. As a result, specific knowledge in these areas is confined largely within the specialties concerned, and, except for the thinnest veneer of information, the body of general medical practitioners remains virtually ignorant of even basic vocabulary and terminology of these disciplines. In my own specialty, I have frequently been impressed by the fact that non-orthopedists are unable to describe fractures properly, and to the end of ameliorating this situation and improving doctor to doctor communication, this monograph is directed.

With the increasing incidence of injuries in this world of high velocity missiles, vehicles, and machinery, it seems that more emphasis should be given to the teaching of management of fractures in the training of a physician, if for no other reason than to expedite referral to the orthopedic surgeon and engender a better understanding of the patient's problems by the referring doctor when the patient returns for continued follow-up care. In addition to securing prompt and proper management of fractures, expediency in accident rooms will be enhanced through better use and understanding of the language of fractures.

As fracture terms are familiar to most physicians, their failure to be used properly probably lies in the medical school programs, where orthopedics is skimmed over very rapidly in order to devote more time to other subjects in the crowded curricula.

The description of fractures depends upon a foundation of fracture terms and a logical presentation of these terms. The language of fractures consists of commonly used words that are part of every physician's vocabulary. However, because of lack of proper orientation and instruction, most physicians have not learned to apply them to clinical situations.

As there is no limit to the number of words one may use to describe a fracture, as long as the terms are accurate, the more words used the more descriptive will be the explanation. It is my intention to simplify the naming of fractures. Thus I have written the book, *The Language of Fractures*, with the desire of producing a textbook small enough and interesting enough to be read from cover to cover, and through it to develop a fracture vocabulary, by gradually adding terms which can be used progressively. The proper use of these descriptive terms will be illustrated by text, photographs, line drawings, and radiographs, and, through repetition, the terms will be assimilated. The book is rich in pictures so as to bring the text to life and thus make a permanent impression on the mind of the reader. As a basic introduction, this book is intended to appeal to medical students, interns, orthopedic residents commencing their training, and all others who are interested in conversing with their friendly orthopedic surgeon.

The book is divided into four sections: (I) a foundation of fracture vocabulary, (II) an application of the vocabulary to specific regions, (III) a bibliography of eponyms, and (IV) a section of fractures that are not fractures, or common pitfalls in the interpretation of fractures. A review appears periodically to allow the reader to reflect on the material covered. Preceding the descriptions in the book will be descriptions of the pertinent anatomy of the region being described, thus giving the student basic insight into the skeletal injury.

Thus if sufficient time and emphasis are not available in the usual medical school curriculum, the student now has a book which may be easily and quickly read and easily and quickly assimilated to enhance his fracture knowledge. As a basic text, it is hoped that this will be a keystone in the development of the physician's knowledge in the discussion and treatment of fractures.

PREFACE FOR 1976 REPRINT

When a book is reprinted the author has the opportunity of re-evaluating what he has written, question whether his original premise proved to be true or whether the book should now be perceived in a different light.

The statements made in 1972 concerning the lack of time available for students in their regular school curriculum would appear more true today than when written.

Although today's research may have uncovered a number of more sophisticated approaches in the surgical end, the basically required knowledge of vocabulary application to specific requirements in knowledge of eponyms and recognition of "non-fractures" would seem a cornerstone on which to build a further medical structure.

My gratification will continue as long as students find the contents meaningful.

ACKNOWLEDGMENTS

In the preparation and publication of this book, I had occasion to call on the talents and efforts of several people without whose assistance it could not have been brought to completion. To Mrs. Sheila Battino for her secretarial help, to Ingram Chodorow for the illustrations, to the Department of Radiology of the Albert Einstein College of Medicine for the use of x-ray films, to Drs. Robert Shimm, Robert Loeffler, Henry Ergas, and Michael Kamelian for their editorial assistance, and to the many medical students and residents at the Albert Einstein affiliated hospitals for constructive criticism and suggestions, I extend my sincerest thanks and profound appreciation.

CONTENTS

1

GENERAL ANATOMY

The skeletal system of man is composed of an articulated series of bones which serve as a rigid supporting and protective framework for the body. Without the support offered by the bones, we would collapse like a glob, and, without their protection, vital organs such as the brain, lungs, and abdominal and pelvic viscera would be extremely v nerable to injury.

In addition, bones serve as levers for muscles, contain marrow which is a factory for red blood cells, and act as the storehouse of calcium and phosphorus.

Bones come in all sizes and shapes and their articulations are also of several varieties. They may be designated as long bones, flat bones, irregular bones, sesamoid bones, and accessory or supernumerary bones.

The gross structure of all bones exists in two forms composed of compact and spongy bony tissue. The compact layer forms the outer shell of the bone and is called the cortex. In long bones, the cortex is thickest toward the middle of the shaft and is thinnest at the ends. The spongy bone, referred to as cancellous bone, occupies the inner aspect of the bone except for a tubular space called the marrow cavity.

Enveloping the cortex of the bone is the periosteum which is a specialized dense fibrous tissue layer containing blood vessels, lymphatics, and nerves.

The endosteum is a thin layer on the inner aspect of the cortex which lines the walls of the marrow cavities and Haversian canals.

Both the periosteum and endosteum have osteogenic properties in young growing individuals, and in response to fractures in children and adults.

Development of Bones

Bone is a specialized type of connective tissue originating from the pluripotential cell mass of primitive mesoderm.

Developmentally, bone forms and grows by two methods: intramembranous and endochondral ossification. Intramembranous ossification occurs by direct metaplasia of the connective tissue precursor into bone. In this method, the mesenchymal cells coalesce to form a fibrous model of the future bone. Ossification then occurs by direct differentiation of the mesenchymal cells into osteoblasts, which proceed to lay down a network of bone trabeculae. This bone deposition expands in all directions to replace the original fibrous model.

In endochondral ossification, however, the mesenchymal cells initially form a cartilage mold of the future bone. Ossification then takes place within the cartilage model by the development of one or more ossific centers called primary and secondary centers of ossification. The pri-

3

mary center is located in the center of the newly developing bone, with the secondary centers of ossification at the ends of the bone. In these regions the preformed cartilage cells pass through several stages resulting in the eventual death of the cartilage cells and replacement by bone (Fig. I.1). The stages of differentiation and ossification of the cartilage cells are as follows: in the center of the bone, in an area called the primary center of ossification, the cartilage cells hypertrophy and arrange themselves in rows. Calcification of the intercellular matrix then occurs, followed by death of the cartilage cells (chondrocytes). Simultaneously, blood vessels with osteoblasts from the peripheral tissues invade the central area. The osteoblasts line the calcified matrix, and new bone is laid down as osteoid. (Osteoid is the uncalcified precursor of bone.) As this is occurring, the calcified cartilage is resorbed, and the new bone that has been laid down is in turn immediately calci-

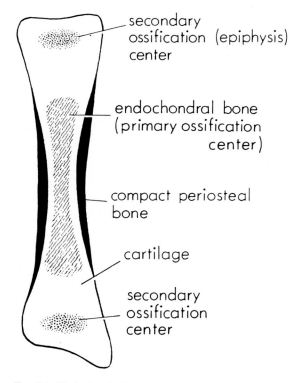

FIG. I.1. Endochondral ossification of a long bone. Long bones are preformed in cartilage with the primary center of ossification starting in the shaft. The epiphyses are the secondary centers of ossification. A periosteal collar surrounds the bone and contributes to its increase in width.

fied. The process of ossification then proceeds centrifugally from the primary center until there has been complete ossification of the cartilage precursor.

During this process, the perichondrium about the periphery of the cartilage mold is transformed into periosteum. The deep layer of the periosteum proceeds to form bone by direct osteogenesis of the intramembranous variety. This periosteal ossification accounts for the increase in thickness of a bone.

Secondary centers of ossification appear at the ends of the bone at various times in skeletal maturation. These centers are separated from the shaft by the epiphyseal plate which is responsible for longitudinal growth. Development and differentiation of the secondary centers into bone is by endochondral ossification.

Classification of Bones

Long bones are those bones whose length is greater than their breadth. Metacarpals, metatarsals, and phalanges, although relatively short, are still considered to be long bones. A long bone has a shaft and two ends, is usually tubular, and is confined to the limbs where it serves as a lever for muscles. The ends of long bones, which are usually covered by articular cartilage are enlarged, thus increasing the surface area of the articulation and affording more stability to the joint.

Developmentally, long bones are preformed in cartilage and their shafts begin to ossify during the 2nd or 3rd fetal month. Their ends (or epiphyses) are secondary centers of ossification and, except for those of the distal femur, proximal tibia, and proximal humerus, are subject to ossification after birth. These latter epiphyses ossify before birth. An exception to the usual long bone formation is the clavicle which has no marrow cavity and is largely preformed in membrane rather than cartilage. The distal phalanges are unique in that they are nonarticular at the distal ends.

Short bones are bones of more cuboidal shape and are found in the carpus and the tarsus. They develop in cartilage and begin to ossify soon after birth. Three short bones, the calcaneous, talus, and cuboid, start to ossify before birth.

It is necessary to know approximately when bones begin to ossify and when their ossification is completed, since fractures occurring in these regions cannot be noted roentgenographically if ossification is not present, and a clinical diagnosis then must be reached solely through physical examination. In addition, mistakes may be made by diagnosing a normal epiphyseal plate as a fracture. Conversely, a fracture may not be noted but be mistaken for a normal epiphyseal plate when the epiphyseal line is already closed. In children it is essential to have comparative films of the opposite extremity to assist with the diagnosis.

Flat bones consist of two layers or plates of compact bone, separated by a thin marrow space, and are mainly preformed in membrane. Most flat bones help form the walls of rounded cavities and are, therefore, curved. The major flat bones to concern the orthopedic surgeon are the sternum, ribs, and scapula.

Irregular bones are bones of mixed shape, namely the vertebrae and those of the pelvis. These are also composed of spongy or cancellous bone within a compact covering similar to flat bones.

Sesamoid bones are bones that develop and are located in certain tendons which glide across the ends of long bones. *The sesamoid bones have no periosteum and have a free surface covered with articular cartilage.* Sesamoid bones serve to improve the angle of approach of a tendon into its insertion, thus increasing the functional efficiency of the joint. There are many sesamoid bones, the most familiar of which are the patella, the pisiform, and the fabella. The fabella occurs in the lateral head of the gastrocnemius muscle and, although classified as such, perhaps is not a true sesamoid according to strict definition of the term, since it has no articular surface and is located in the belly of a muscle.

Accessory or supernumerary bones are bones that develop from separate centers of ossification. These centers, over a period of time, may obtain bony union with the parent bone. Where one or more of these centers have failed to fuse or unite with the main mass of bone, it remains as a small discrete ossicle located adjacent to the particular parent bone. These bones occasionally cause difficulty in radiographic diagnosis of fractures and need to be recognized (Part IV, page 332). Usually, however, they are bilateral so that comparative x-rays of the other extremity may aid in the correct diagnosis.

CLASSIFICATION OF FRACTURES

Definition of Fractures

To understand fractures, we must start at the beginning.

A *fracture* is a complete or incomplete break in the continuity of bone or cartilage. This pertains despite the shape of the bone, be it long, flat, or irregular in contour. Thus it becomes obvious that the word fracture must be further amplified by various descriptive terms.

Fractures may be caused by direct or indirect trauma, according to whether the forces are applied directly to the bone involved or at a distance from the affected bone and transmitted to it.

Fracture forces may be compressing, torsional, shearing, or occur by tension, and may cause fractures through normal bone by a single major trauma or by repeated low intensity stresses or fatigue. Fractures may also occur through diseased bone after minimal trauma.

A *complete fracture* is one where both cortices of the bone have been broken as opposed to an *incomplete fracture* where only one cortex has been broken (Fig. I.2). If a fracture contains more than two fragments, it is classified as a *comminuted fracture*.

Closed Fracture (Simple Fracture)

A *closed* or *simple fracture* is one in which the skin and soft tissues overlying the fracture are intact and there is no communication with the outside environment.

Open Fracture (Compound Fracture)

An *open* or *compound fracture* exists anytime the fracture site communicates with the outside environment (Fig. I.3). This is true whether the wound or skin defect is a small pinhole, puncture wound, or massive

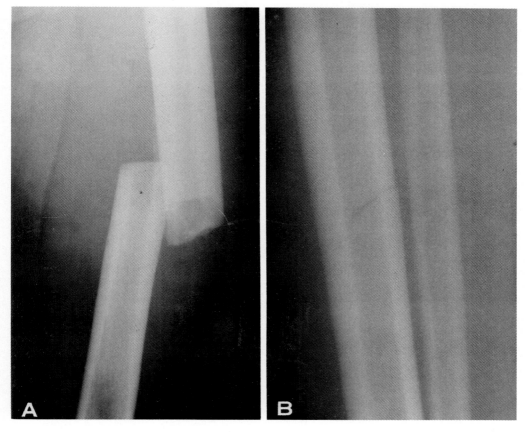

Fig. I.2.
(A) Complete fracture. The fracture has passed through both cortices of the bone.
(B) Incomplete fracture. Note that the fracture extends only through the posterior cortex of the tibia; the anterior cortex has remained intact.

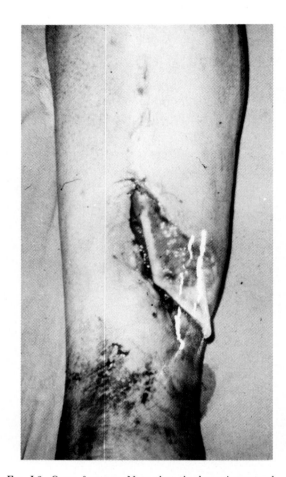

FIG. I.3. Open fracture. Note that the bone is protruding through the skin and thus communicating with the outside environment.

soft tissue loss; whether the wound is relatively clean or grossly contaminated; or whether the skin defect is caused by the bone perforating the skin from within, or the defect is caused by a missile or fracturing agent entering from without (Fig. I.4).

Compound fractures are considered by the orthopedic surgeon to be surgical emergencies because of the contamination and the possibility of infection, and thus treatment must be instituted immediately. Innocent looking puncture wounds may and have been responsible for death from gas gangrene or a persistent chronic bone infection (osteomyelitis). The object of early therapy is to effect debridement with a resultant clean wound, the restoration of fracture position being only of secondary importance.

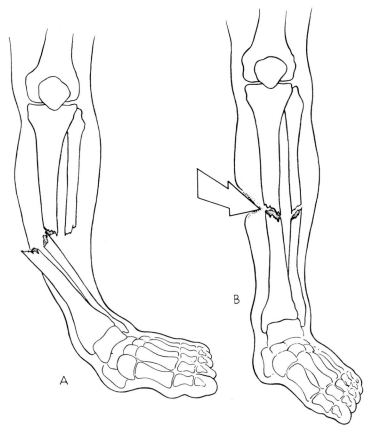

Fig. I.4.

(A) Compound fracture caused by an inside-out injury. The skin defect is caused, following the fracture, by the bone perforating the skin from within.

(B) Outside-in compound fracture. In this injury, the skin defect is produced by the fracturing agent entering from without.

Thus once the skin is broken, any fracture which has been exposed to the outside environment is a compound fracture.

If a soft tissue defect communicates with a segment of bone but not with the fracture site, it is *not* considered to be a compound fracture.

Open reduction by surgery converts closed fractures to open ones. Although these surgically elective procedures are performed under sterile conditions, they are not without risk of infection.

ESTABLISHING THE LOCATION OF FRACTURE REFERENCE POINTS

To describe the location of a fracture, points of reference must be established. These may be standard anatomic reference points, such as the medial malleolus, surgical neck of the humerus, medial femoral condyle, and base of metacarpal, or, as will now be described, arbitrarily designated.

Regardless of the size or shape, the shafts of long bones can be divided into thirds: namely proximal, middle, and distal (Fig. I.5). Thus any fracture in these bones can be described as a fracture occurring through the proximal, middle, or distal third.

The points of junction of these segments are referred to as the junction of the proximal and middle third and the junction of the middle and distal third. Fractures at these levels are referred to as fractures at the junction of the proximal and middle third (PM3) and junction of middle and distal third (MD3). A lesion occurring at or about the midpoint of the bone, although located in the middle third, may be referred to as a midshaft fracture.

Thus fractures of the shafts of long bones are said to be located in the proximal, middle, or distal thirds or at their junctions (Fig. I.6).

The location of lesions in other areas may be described by their anatomic location, such as a fracture of the medial malleolus, fracture of the surgical neck of the humerus, fracture of the patella, and fracture of the superior pubic ramus. Further consideration of anatomic reference points will be considered in the section on specific fractures.

DIRECTION OF FRACTURE LINES

Now that we have established terminology as to the location or level of a fracture, we can continue to supplement our fracture vocabulary by describing the direction of the fracture. This is best achieved by noting the relation of the fracture to the long axis of the bone in the case of long bones, and the cortices in the case of irregular bones. The direction of a fracture may be transverse, oblique, spiral, or comminuted.

Transverse Fracture

A transverse fracture is one that occurs when the fracture line is at

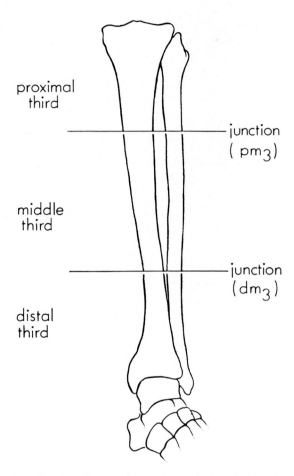

proximal
third

middle
third

distal
third

junction
(pm₃)

junction
(dm₃)

FIG. I.5. Despite the shape of various long bones, the shaft may be divided into proximal, middle, and distal thirds. The points of junction are referred to as the junction of the proximal and middle third and middle and distal third.

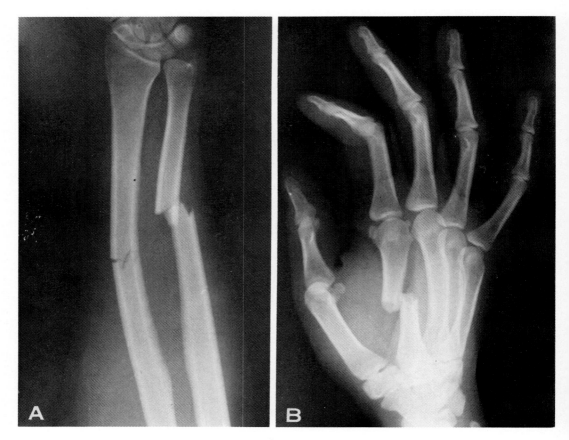

FIG. I.6.
(A) Closed fracture of the middle third of the radius and the junction of middle and distal third of the ulna.
(B) Closed complete fracture of the midshaft of the second metacarpal.

right angles to the cortices or long axis of the bone, whether the bone be long or irregular in shape. Transverse fractures may be complete or incomplete, open or closed, and may occur at any location.

Therefore, any fracture which is transverse can be easily recognized and stated to occur in the bone involved at a specific level.

In the diagram and radiographs, we see that we now can amplify a fracture description by designating the direction, location, completeness, and nature of the fracture (Fig. I.7). For example, one may see a closed, complete transverse fracture of the distal third of the radius and ulna (Fig. I.7D).

Oblique Fracture

An oblique fracture is one in which the fracture line runs obliquely to the long axis of the bone or cortices. Again, the location and the completeness, as well as the other features, can be described (Fig. I.8).

Spiral Fracture

A spiral fracture is caused by a torsional force and is somewhat like a long oblique fracture that spans a greater area and encircles the shaft of the long bone, thus forming a spiral in relation to the long axis of the bone (Fig. I.9).

Comminuted Fracture

A comminuted fracture is one that has more than two fracture fragments. This holds true whether the number is three, three thousand, or three million, and regardless of location. Thus, at any time and in any location, if a fracture has more than two fragments, it is considered comminuted (Fig. I.10).

There are specific types of comminuted fractures which, because of their appearance, have been given specific names (*e.g.*, a comminuted fracture with butterfly fragment and segmental fractures).

A *butterfly fragment* is a wedge-shaped fragment, split off from the main fragments.

Segmental fractures are those in which the fracture divides the long bone into several segments (Fig. I.11).

A pitfall one may encounter occurs when an oblique fracture, on x-ray, is observed straight on. In this case it will look like a comminuted fracture; however, a second view at right angles to the first will demonstrate the obliquity of the fracture (Fig. I.12).

Review

We may pause for a few minutes to reflect on our vocabulary to this point. A fracture is described by the bone involved and its location within the bone, whether it is complete or incomplete, open or closed, and by the direction of the fracture line. For review, identify the fractures demonstrated in the radiographs (Figs. I.A–I.D) (see page 385 for correct identification.)

OTHER DESCRIPTIVE TERMS

To augment the descriptions of fractures, further terminology can be employed.

Distraction

Distraction occurs when the apposing ends of the fracture fragments are kept apart. This may be the result of excessive traction caused by the pull of tendons, or by the use of too much weight in fracture treat-

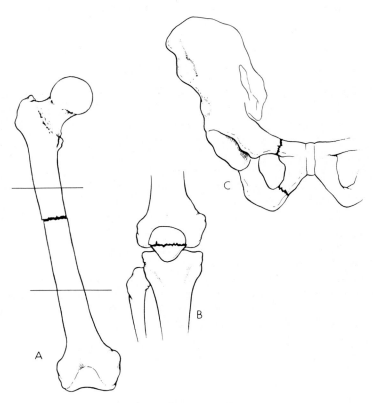

Fig. I.7. Transverse fractures.
(A) Transverse fracture of the middle third of the femur.
(B) Transverse fracture of the midpatella.
(C) Transverse fracture of the superior and inferior pubic rami.

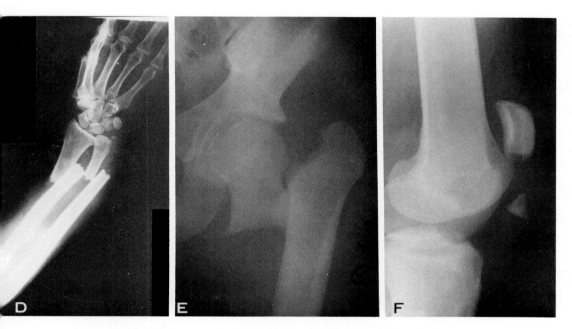

(D) Closed transverse fracture of the distal third of the radius and ulna.
(E) Transverse fracture of the neck of the femur.
(F) Transverse fracture of distal third of the patella.

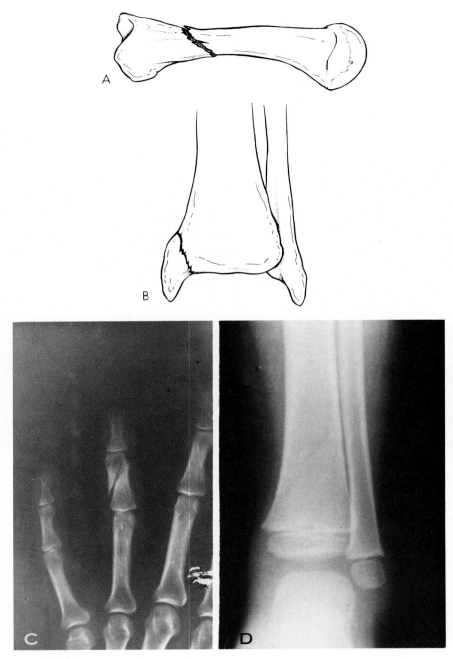

FIG. I.8. Oblique fractures.

(A) Oblique fracture of the proximal third of a metacarpal.

(B) Oblique fracture of the medial malleolus.

(C) Closed oblique fracture involving the middle and distal third of the middle phalanx.

(D) Closed incomplete oblique fracture of the distal third of the tibia.

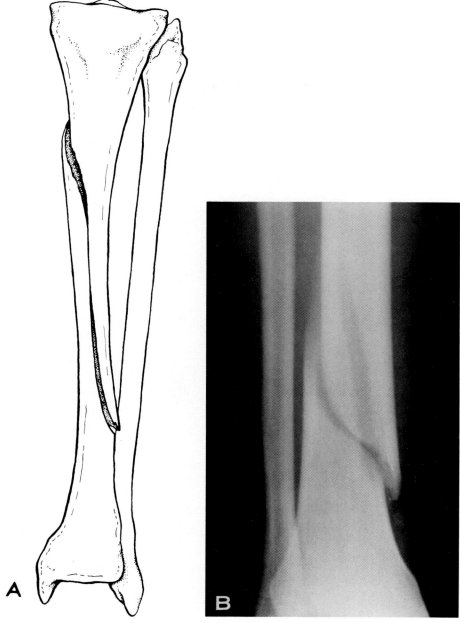

FIG. I.9. Spiral fractures.
(A) Spiral fracture of the middle third of the tibia.
(B) Radiograph of a closed spiral fracture of the distal third of the tibia.

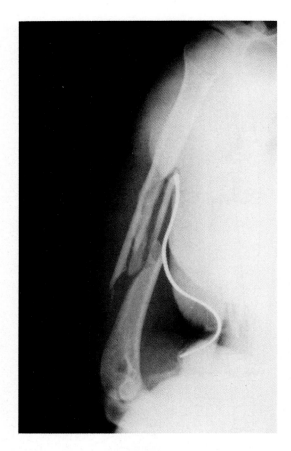

FIG. I.10. Comminuted fracture of the middle third of the humerus. Note that there are more than two fragments.

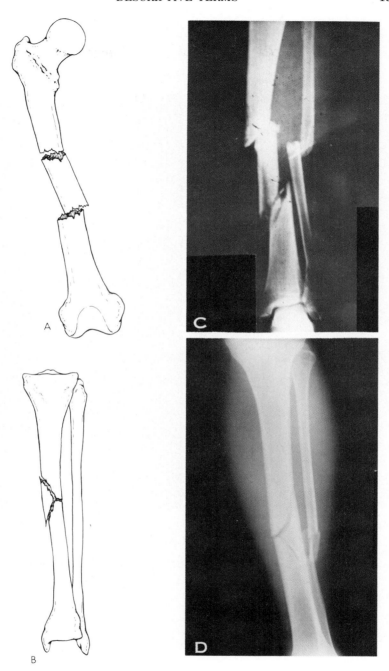

FIG. I.11.
    (A) Diagrammatic representation of a segmental fracture of the femur.
    (B) Diagrammatic representation of a butterfly fragment.
    (C) Segmental fracture of the tibia.
    (D) Butterfly fragment of the middle third of the tibia.

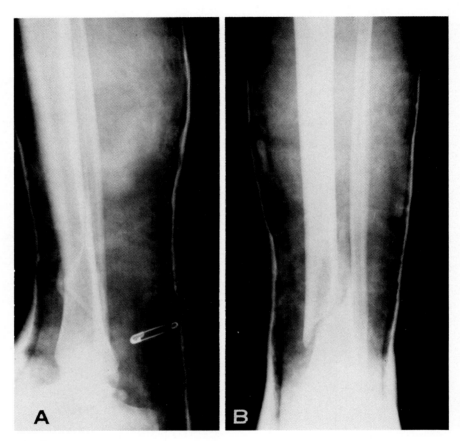

Fɪɢ. I.12.

(A) On lateral view the fracture appears to be comminuted with a butterfly fragment involving the distal third of the tibia.

(B) View at right angles (anteroposterior) demonstrates the oblique nature of the fracture and the absence of comminution.

REVIEW FIGURES I.A–I.D

Fig. I.A

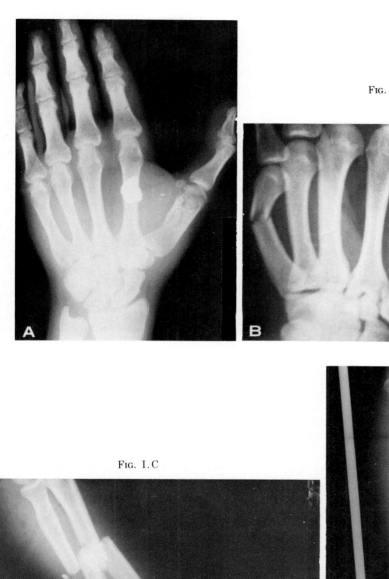

Fig. I.B

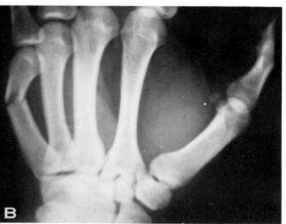

Fig. I.D

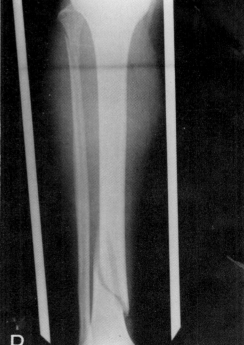

Fig. I.C

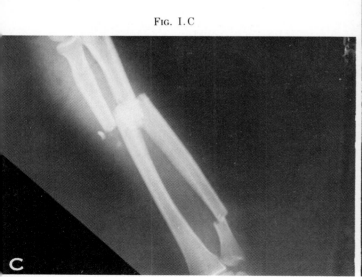

ment. The fracture may also be kept apart by interposed soft tissues between the fragments (as ligaments, muscles, tendons, periosteum, or foreign bodies), or may even occur following fixation of a bone when bony reabsorption occurs at the fracture site during fracture healing (Fig. I.13). As fracture healing is concerned with osteoblastic activity and these cells creep and do not jump, distraction is an unhealthy situation for fracture healing.

Impaction

Impaction occurs when one fragment of bone is forcibly driven or telescoped into the adjacent fragment, or when the fracture fragments are allowed to press forcibly against each other. Impaction usually occurs in an area of cancellous bone, since its spongy nature permits the compression necessary to effect impaction (Fig. I.14). With impaction, a degree of natural stability is produced. Fracture healing is concerned with osteoblastic activity, which, as noted previously, progresses across fracture surfaces by creeping subsitution. Thus with stability produced and the extremely close contact of bony surfaces, impaction is advantageous for fracture healing.

Impaction can also occur in areas of cortical bone; however, here the fragments are not telescoped. Instead, the fracture fragments are pressed tightly against each other. This type of compression or impaction is effected surgically with fixation devices which allow compressing forces to be applied against the bone ends.

Specific types of fractures within the description of impaction are depression fractures and compression fractures.

Depression Fractures

One form of impaction is depression. A depression fracture occurs when the hard surface of one bone is driven into the relatively softer surface of another, and, as a result, the peripheral part of the bone receiving the force is pushed into the softer underlying cancellous bone. This most commonly occurs in the area of the knee when the hard femoral condyle is driven into the softer tibial plateau, depressing the articular surface of the plateau into the underlying cancellous bone (Fig. I.15).

Compression Fractures

Another form of impaction occurs in the form of compression. This is most commonly seen in the body of vertebrae. Here, by forceful flexion of the vertebral column, the superior and inferior surfaces of the vertebral body are driven toward each other and impaction or compression occurs, producing a wedge-shaped vertebra (Fig. I.16).

Avulsion Fractures

Bony prominences often serve as attachments for muscles, ligaments, and tendons. These areas are vulnerable to fracture by either the dy-

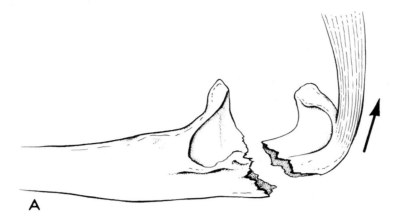

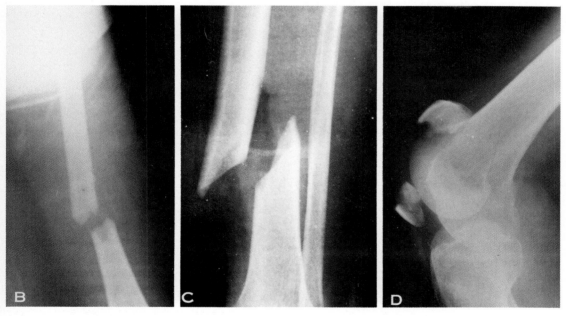

Fig. I.13. Distraction.

(A) Diagrammatic representation of distraction. Note how the pull of the triceps keeps the fragments apart.

(B) Distraction of a closed transverse fracture of the femur due to excessive traction during treatment.

(C) Distraction of an open spiral fracture of the middle and distal third of the tibia, the fragments being kept apart by the skin and other interposed soft tissues.

(D) Transverse fracture of the midpatella with comminution of the distal half. Distraction is due to pull of quadriceps muscles.

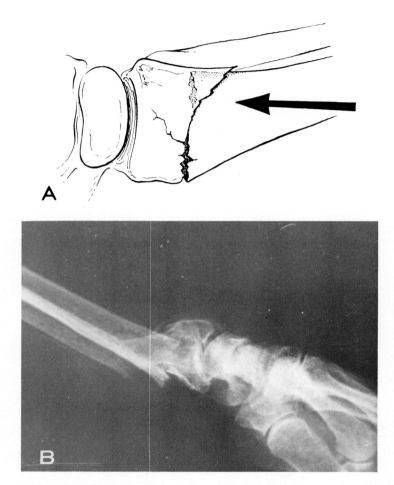

Fig. I.14 (A and B). Impaction. Telescoping of the proximal fragment into the distal fragment in an area of cancellous bone has resulted in an impacted fracture of the distal third of the radius.

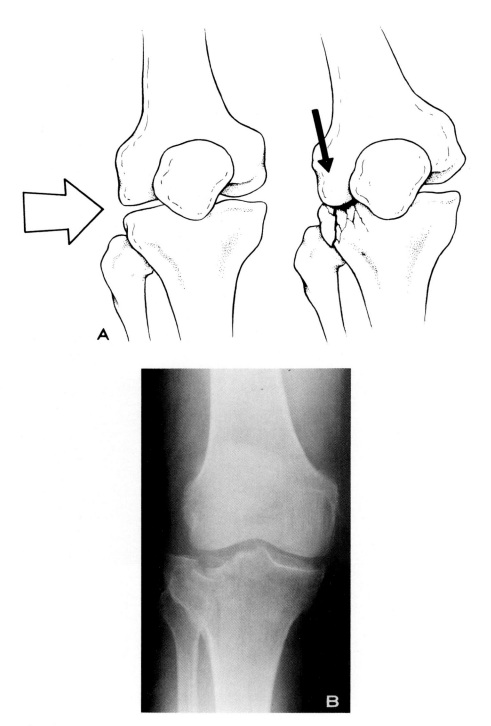

Fɪɢ. I.15. Depression fracture of the tibia.

(A) Fracture of the tibial plateau has occurred as a result of the hard femoral condyle being driven into the relatively softer tibial plateau.

(B) One can note the increased density beneath the articular surface of the tibial plateau which is composed of the compressed cancellous bone plus the denser subchondral bone.

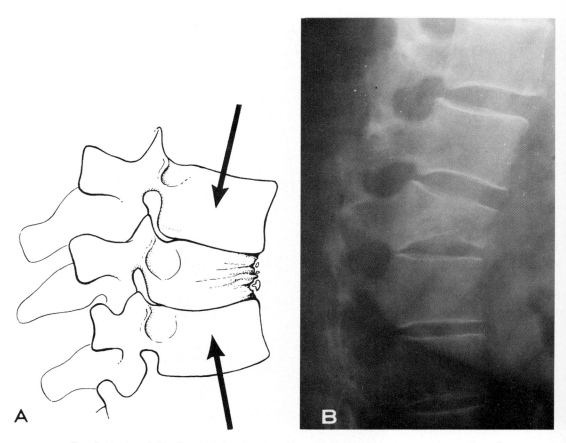

Fig. I.16 (A and B). Compression fracture. Forceful flexion forces cause compression of the anterior aspect of the vertebrae by driving the superior and inferior surfaces of the vertebral body toward each other.

namic pull of a forcibly contracting muscle or the resistive force of a strong ligament. Violent contraction of a muscle can cause rupture of the muscle belly or its tendon, or can pull away a fragment of bone at the insertion of the tendon. At ligamentous insertions, violent trauma applied in a direction which places the ligament under great tension may avulse a fragment of bone rather than rupture the ligament. This, for example, occurs with twisting injuries to the ankle.

Thus an avulsion fracture occurs when fragments of bone are pulled away from their original position by an active contraction of a muscle or the passive resistance of a ligament against a force in the opposite direction.

Avulsion fractures, like other fractures, are classified as to location of the fracture, the direction of the fracture line, whether they are open or closed, or whether they are comminuted or not. Needless to say, avulsion fractures are usually distracted (Fig. I.17).

Intraarticular Fractures

An intraarticular fracture is a fracture which extends into and involves an articular surface of a joint (Fig. I.18). These fractures may or may not be displaced, and the amount of joint surface involved has no bearing on the nomenclature. The fracture may be a simple hairline fracture with no displacement, or the joint can be severely involved with disruption of the entire articular surface. Avulsion fractures very commonly affect joint surfaces and can involve only a small part of the articular surface or constitute a large fragment.

Incomplete Fractures

Incomplete fractures occur when only one cortex of the bone has been broken. Incomplete fractures are relatively stable and, if protected (so that no subsequent stresses are placed upon them), will tend to maintain their position indefinitely. Incomplete fractures are common in short bones, irregularly shaped bones, and flat bones. There are certain incomplete fractures which occur exclusively in children, probably because of the elasticity of their bones. These are greenstick fractures and torus fractures which will be discussed subsequently under "Fractures in Children" (see "Greenstick Fracture," page 52 and "Torus Fracture," page 52).

FRACTURES DUE TO BONY ALTERATION

Pathologic Fractures

Pathologic fractures are those fractures occurring in a bone which has been weakened by a disease process. The basic pathology which produces the proclivity to fracture may be the result of local bone changes or the result of a systemic process which affects the entire skeleton.

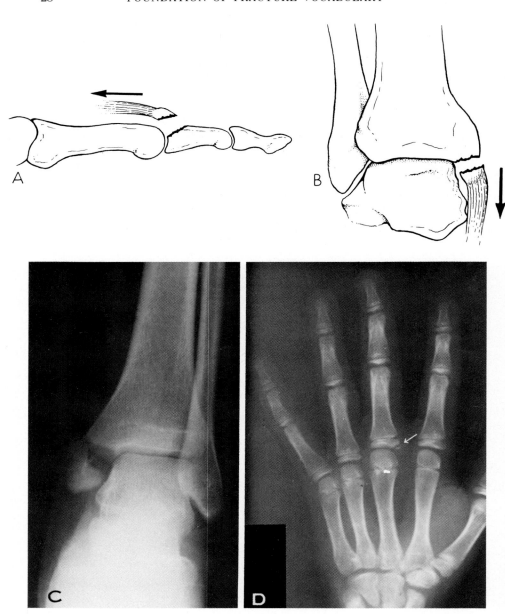

Fig. I.17.

(A) Avulsion fracture at the base of the dorsal surface of the middle phalanx.

(B) Transverse avulsion fracture of the medial malleolus.

(C) Transverse avulsion fracture of the medial malleolus. Note that the fracture fragments are distracted.

(D) Avulsion fracture of the base of the epiphysis of the proximal phalanx of the middle finger.

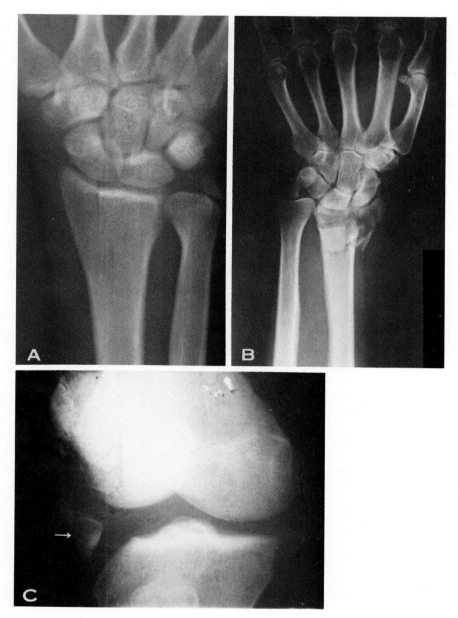

FIG. I.18. Intraarticular fractures.
 (A) Incomplete, nondisplaced intraarticular fracture of the distal radius.
 (B) More extensive fracture involving the articular surface of the distal radius.
 (C) Intraarticular avulsion fracture of a proximal tibial plateau.

Either may produce a defect in the cortical structure of the bone with a resultant zone of weakness. Thus, depending upon the cause of the deficiency, pathologic fractures may be classified as those due to local bone changes or those due to generalized skeletal disease.

Local changes may be secondary to infection; benign, malignant, or metastatic tumors; or disuse, whereas systemic diseases may be either congenital in origin or acquired. Examples of congenital generalized skeletal disease are osteogenesis imperfecta and osteopetrosis. Acquired generalized skeletal diseases include rickets, osteomalacia, osteoporosis, scurvy, and Paget's disease.

For our purposes, it should be noted that these fractures are described similarly to other fractures as to direction, location, completeness, position, and alignment, with the additional note that the fracture has taken place through diseased bone (Fig. I.19).

Frequently, the diagnosis of the pathologic process is not made until, for an unrelated reason, an x-ray is obtained and the diseased bone recognized. On the other hand, previous knowledge of the congenital or systemic diseases allows for ready recognition.

There are certain features which may lead one to suspect that a pathologic fracture has occurred, even in the absence of clear roentgenographic evidence. These are:

1. A history of congenital or acquired bone disease.
2. A fracture that has been caused with minimal stress.
3. A fracture line which is often transverse in nature.
4. Pain or discomfort preceding the fracture episode.

Additional laboratory tests or even tissue biopsy may be necessary to confirm or rule out the diagnosis of a pathologic fracture and the treatment, depends upon the underlying disease.

An important consideration in pathologic fractures is the predisposition of the bone to additional fractures. Prolonged treatment of the initial fracture would be determined by the knowledge as to whether the disease is localized or generalized. In the case of malignant or metastatic tumors, the static or progressive nature of the disease also will determine the type of management.

Stress Fracture (Fatigue Fracture)

A fatigue or stress fracture is the result of repeated, relatively trivial, trauma to an otherwise normal bone. It occurs not as a sudden break in bony continuity but as the result of alteration of the bone in the form of gradual local dissolution, secondary to repeated minor and usually unaccustomed insults. This may or may not result in a complete fracture.

Bone is quite sensitive to the amount of stress imposed upon it and both lack of stress and excessive stress result in local change in the form of resorption. In a fatigue fracture, the repeated stresses produce such resorption. If the stress is discontinued, the process may be ar-

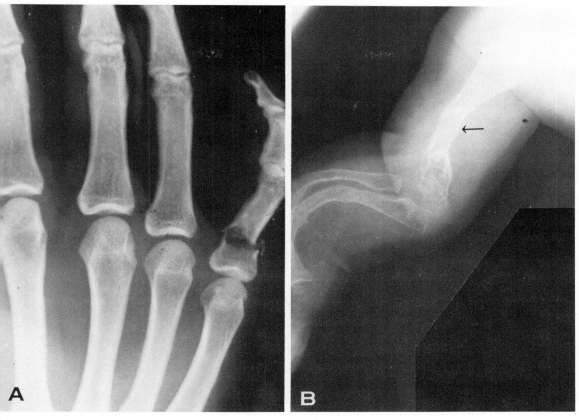

Fig. I.19.

(A) Pathologic transverse fracture at the junction of the proximal and middle third of the proximal phalanx. This lesion occurred through a bone cyst of the small finger.

(B) Pathologic transverse fracture of the humerus in a patient with osteogenesis imperfecta. Note the severe deformity of the bones as a result of the many fractures.

rested, but, if it persists, a fracture may occur through this weakened region.

Fatigue fractures occur most frequently in the lower extremities, especially the metatarsals, and only rarely in the upper extremities. These fractures are found most commonly in military recruits who are subjected to unaccustomed vigorous activities in the form of marching and jumping. They are not limited to military personnel, however; the unconditioned athlete, the new door-to-door salesman, or the weekend physical fitness enthusiast may all develop fatigue fractures. The term has, in the past, generally been used to refer to fractures of the metatarsals associated with the prolonged walking, marching, or running. Similar fractures may occur in other bones, however, as the pelvis, calcaneus, tibia, fibula, and femoral neck and shaft. Because the fracture is less well known in these regions, it may often go unrecognized. By establishing the fracture reference point and noting the direction of the fracture, these injuries may be easily described.

The phenomenon of fatigue fractures may be readily understood when one considers the fact that the plaster can be chipped from a wall, either by a single heavy blow of a hammer or by tapping the wall lightly and repeatedly.

Review

Let us again pause to reflect on our vocabulary. In addition to the nature, location, and direction of a fracture, the description may be further augmented by terms as distraction, impaction, and avulsion. Joint involvement may be described as well as pathologic and stress conditions.

For review, describe the fractures shown in the radiographs (Figs. I.E–I.H). See page 385 for correct identification.

POSITION AND ALIGNMENT

It is imperative in the description of fractures to describe the relationship of the fragments to one another. This is usually done by describing the position of the distal fragment in relation to the proximal one. Several terms are needed to express this relationship.

Alignment

Alignment is the relationship of the longitudinal axis of one fragment to another. Deviation of alignment or malalignment is the result of angulation of the fracture fragments (Fig. I.20).

Position

Position is the relationship of the fragments to their normal anatomical structure. Loss of position is called displacement and may result from the loss of apposition, overriding, or rotation. In the shafts of long bones various combinations can occur. For example, fracture fragments may be displaced yet well aligned, or may be angulated or rotated with little displacement.

Therefore, we should consider the various combinations (Fig. I.21). First of all, a fracture may be in good position and alignment. In other words, there is no displacement or disturbance of the bone from its normal anatomical structure, and no angulation. Secondly, the fracture may be angulated or malaligned with relatively no displacement. In this situation, some apposition or contact of the ends of the fragment is present. Thirdly, a fracture may be completely displaced and still be in good alignment. Here, overriding has occurred but the bony fragments are parallel to each other. This type of fragment relationship can be referred to as "bayonet apposition." A fracture may have rotary dis-

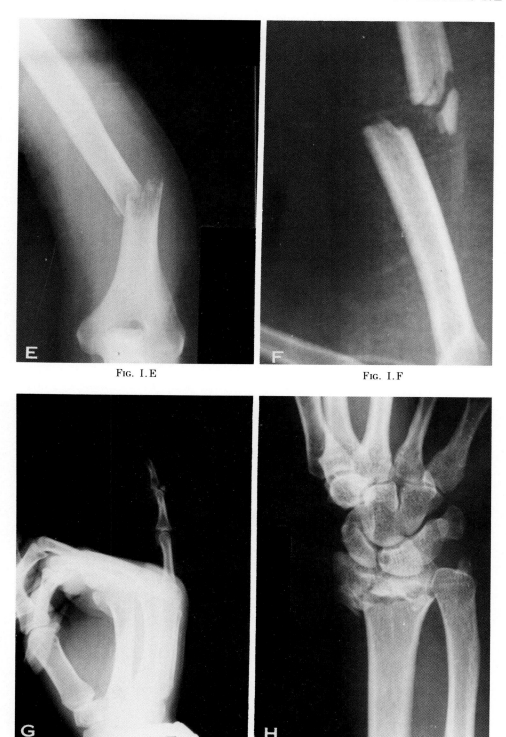

FIG. I.E

FIG. I.F

FIG. I.G

FIG. I.H

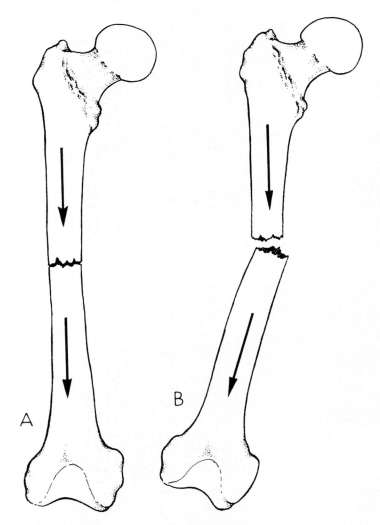

Fig. I.20. Alignment is the relationship of the longitudinal axis of one fragment to another.

(A) Good alignment.

(B) Angulation of the longitudinal axis of one fragment to the other and thus malalignment.

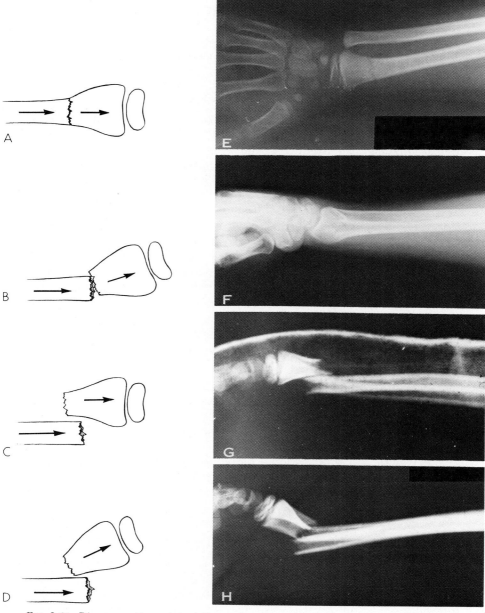

Fig. I.21. Diagrammatic representation and radiographs of the position and alignment of a transverse fracture of the distal radius.

(A) Good position and alignment. Note there is no disturbance from the normal anatomical position.

(B) Similar fracture which is angulated but relatively nondisplaced.

(C) Transverse fracture of the distal radius which is displaced, however, in good alignment. Note there is no angulation despite significant displacement.

(D) Shows the same fracture, angulated and displaced.

(E) Transverse fracture of the distal radius in good position and alignment.

(F) Transverse fracture of the distal radius which is angulated but relatively nondisplaced.

(G) Displaced fracture without angulation (bayonet apposition).

(H) Fracture which is both angulated and displaced.

placement and also still be in good alignment. Finally, a fracture may be displaced and angulated, in which case overriding and angulation have occurred.

Direction of Angulation

The description of the direction of angulation is often the source of confusion! The direction of angulation can be described (1) by the direction of angular displacement of the distal fragment in relation to the proximal fragment or (2) by the direction of the apex of the angle formed by the fracture fragments. Most often the direction of angulation is confused with the direction of angular displacement of the distal fragment. Too often, for example, a Colles' fracture is said to have dorsal angulation when dorsal angular displacement of the distal fragment is meant. Because of this, it seems more rational to establish a principle and describe direction of the distal fragment in relation to the proximal one; however, since both methods are in common usage, both will be presented. Thus if the apex of the fractured radius is volar, this is called either volar angulation of the fracture or dorsal angular displacement of the distal fragment, and, in similar fashion, if a fractured tibia has its apex medially, this is called medial angulation of the fracture or lateral angular displacement of the distal fragment (Fig. I.22).

REDUCTION OF FRACTURES

Once a fracture has occurred and the fragments displaced, an attempt must be made to restore the fracture fragments to their normal anatomic position. This procedure is known as reduction of a fracture. Reduction may be accomplished in two ways:

1. *Closed reductions.* Closed reductions are reductions of fractures which do not require an operative incision to be made. This type of reduction is produced by traction or manipulation of the fracture fragments, or a combination of both.
2. *Open reductions.* An open reduction is a restoration of the fracture fragments through surgical exposure of the fracture site.

Fixation

Fixation is the method of holding the fracture fragments in position following reduction. Fixation may be performed by (1) external means, such as cast immobilization, and (2) by internal means. Obviously for fixation to be internal, operative or open reduction must have occurred; however, not all open reductions require internal fixation.

Internal fixation may be accomplished by using devices of various types, for example, screws which cross the fracture line, plates which lie on the outer surface of the bone, or intramedullary fixation in which a rod is inserted into the medullary canal (Fig. I.23). Frequently internal fixation also requires external immobilization. Thus fractures may be said to have open reduction with internal fixation, open reduction and

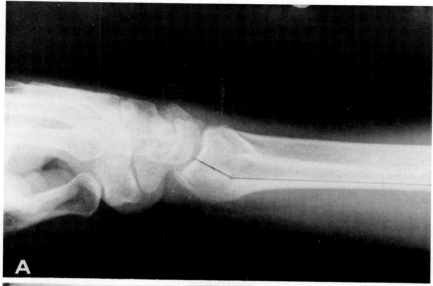

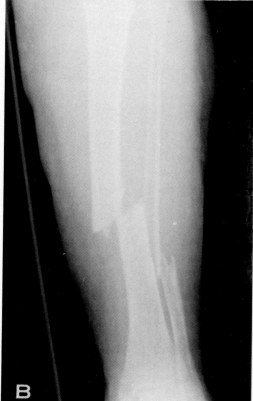

Fig. I.22.

(A) Transverse fracture of the distal radius with dorsal angular deformity of the distal fragment or volar angulation of the fracture.

(B) Oblique comminuted fracture of the middle third of the tibia and junction of middle and distal third of the fibula, with lateral angulation of the distal fragment or medial angulation of the fracture.

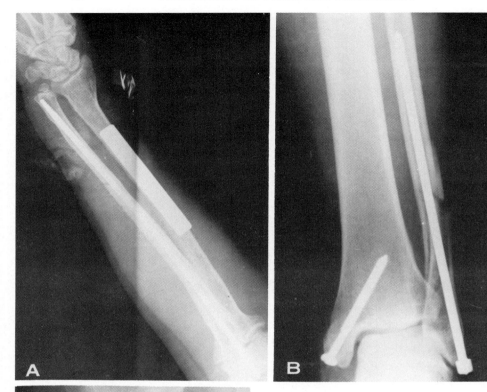

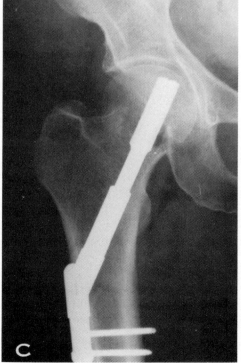

FIG. I.23. Forms of internal fixation.

(A) Internal fixation has been used to immobilize a fracture of both bones of the forearm. A bone plate has been placed on the radius and an intramedullary rod placed into the ulna.

(B) Screw placed across the fracture of the medial malleolus and an intramedullary screw in the fibula.

(C) Intracapsular hip fracture fixed with a hip nail and side plate.

external fixation, a combination of the two, or closed reduction and external fixation.

FRACTURE HEALING

The onset of the healing of fractures begins shortly after the fracture occurs. The mechanism of healing, however, is not a uniform procedure as there are basic differences in the healing of fractures in cortical bone, cancellous bone, and bone that has been placed under compression and rigid fixation by means of surgical techniques. Although it is not within the scope of this book to explore the intricate details of fracture healing, the basic principles should be mentioned.

Fracture Healing of Cortical Bone

Fractures in cortical bone heal by the formation of new bone which tends to bridge the fracture gap between the bone fragments. This new

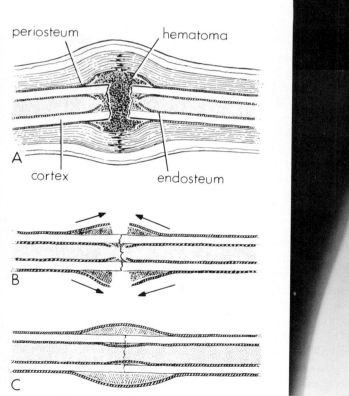
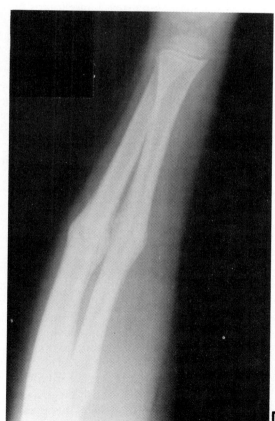

FIG. I.24. Fracture healing in cortical bone.

(A) Following a fracture, there is rupture of the periosteum and endosteum, and formation of a hematoma at the fracture site.

(B) Periosteal and endosteal response results in bone deposition which proceeds toward the fracture.

(C) A collar of callus eventually surrounds the fracture.

(D) Radiograph of provisional callus surrounding the fracture. Note the fracture line is still visible in the center.

bone is called callus, which is a complex structure composed of fibrous tissue, blood vessels, cartilage, and bone.

The process of fracture healing in cortical bone is a composite one in which ossification passes through several stages: hematoma formation, formation and organization of granulation tissue, development of provisional callus, formation of secondary callus, and remodeling. These stages proceed by a reaction of the periosteum and the endosteum, and with organization and ossification of the fracture hematoma.

Initially following the fracture, there is rupture of the periosteum and endosteum, in addition to injury to the surrounding soft tissues. As a result, a hematoma is formed at the fracture site which contains, in addition to blood, the tissue debris of bone and soft tissue, and living and dead bone cells. Subsequently, the hematoma becomes organized as there is an ingrowth of blood vessels, accompanied by inflammatory cells and fibroblasts forming granulation tissue. Shortly thereafter, young, immature bone is laid down about the blood vessels, arranging itself in a haphazard pattern.

The fibroblasts, under the influence of unknown factors, differentiate into osteoblasts and chondroblasts, and subsequently lead to the formation of osteoid tissue which is then mineralized. This process of differentiation may occur by direct metaplasia of fibroblast to osteoblast and formation of new bone proceeding in the manner of intramembranous ossification, or there can be differentiation into chondroblasts with the formation of cartilage and later followed by bone formation in the manner of endochondral ossification.

The participation of the periosteum in fracture healing is of major importance. The periosteum is composed of two layers, an outer layer of dense fibrous tissue, and an inner cambium layer, which, in young growing individuals, is made up of proliferating osteoblasts. In the adult, this inner layer is indistinguishable from dense connective tissue; however, in response to fracture, it reverts back to a layer of proliferating osteoblasts.

The contribution of the periosteum occurs in response to the fracture as the osteoblasts which are present in the cambium layer begin to proliferate rapidly. This rapid proliferation leads to a deposition of new bone, initially at a distance of several millimeters away on either side of the fracture. This new bone deposition then proceeds to expand toward the site of the fracture and eventually links up to form a collar of external callus that surrounds each fragment. Similarly, the endosteal lining of the bone, when it is torn after a fracture, responds by active proliferation, replacing the bone marrow with new bone, which subsequently bridges the fracture. Thus through these three elements (the hematoma, the periosteum, and the endosteum) we have the formation of primary immature bone, also referred to as woven or fiber bone (Fig. I.24).

Secondary callus is then formed upon the surface of the primary bone. In response to the stresses of normal function, the random pattern of the immature bone is then rearranged to the more regular pattern of mature bone. This process occurs as the primary callus is removed by resorptive activity of the osteoclasts while bone deposition is occurring due to the osteogenic activity of the osteoblasts. This new bone, however, is formed along lines of stress, producing a lamellar pattern.

Eventually excessive new bone is resorbed, and, via remodeling, the natural contour of the bone is restored.

Fracture Healing of Cancellous Bone

Fractures occurring through areas of cancellous bone unite with little or no callus formation. Here osteosynthesis or fracture healing occurs by direct osteoblastic bridging (creeping substitution) and thus there must be direct contact of the fragment ends. If direct bony contact cannot be achieved and a gap exists, the space is occupied by a hematoma followed by the steps leading to callus formation.

Fracture Healing Associated with Compression and Rigid Fixation

Recently techniques of fracture treatment with rigid fixation and compression have been developed, and fracture healing without callus formation has been demonstrated. With compression, the fracture defect is bridged directly by osteogenic cells with little or no periosteal reaction. Vascular channels have also been demonstrated to directly cross the fracture line (Fig. I.25). In addition to direct bony bridging,

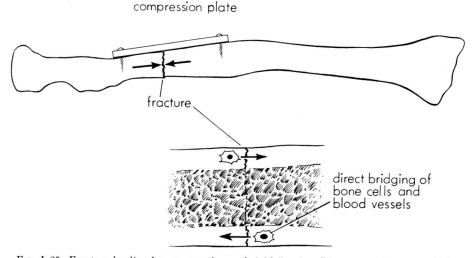

Fig. I.25. Fracture healing by compression and rigid fixation. Diagrammatic representation of direct bridging of osteogenic cells and blood vessels.

there is also immediate remodeling, as bone formation, deposition and resorption occur simultaneously as a result of osteoblastic and osteoclastic activity.

TERMS RELATED TO FRACTURE UNION

In addition to the differences in the mechanism of union, other factors affect the rate and quality of fracture healing. These are: the age of the patient, the general health and nutrition of the patient, the presence or absence of systemic or local infection or generalized or local bone disease, the severity of the trauma, the location of the fracture, the rigidity of the fixation, the quality of the reduction, and the regional blood supply. Generally, the greater the surface area involved in the fracture, the better the healing and, the larger the bone, the longer the time required for healing.

Union is the final goal in the treatment of all fractures. There are, however, some deviations of this normal process of bone healing that will be described.

Delayed Union

Delayed union exists when a fracture fails to unite in the time usually required for union to take place. The period of time for bone to unite varies in different individuals, in different anatomical locations, and under different circumstances.

In delayed union, fracture repair, although retarded, is proceeding and will eventually produce firm union provided additional adverse stresses are not added.

The causes of delayed union are inadequate or interrupted immobilization, unsatisfactory reduction, severe local trauma, circulatory compromise, infection, or separation of fragments due to distraction or loss of bone substance.

Slow Union

There are many fractures that even under ideal conditions are known to heal slowly. However, if this rate of union is normal or average for a particular fracture, location, and age group, etc., the fracture can be considered to be undergoing slow union. Most importantly slow union is not to be confused with delayed union, which is retarded healing beyond the normal rate for a given fracture.

Nonunion

Nonunion exists when there is failure of union of the fracture fragments and the processes of bone repair have ceased completely. All the factors that cause delayed union, if allowed to persist or are enhanced, will cause nonunion. With nonunion, the apposing ends of the fracture fragments become atrophic, and the medullary canals occluded, being covered over by sclerotic, eburnated bone.

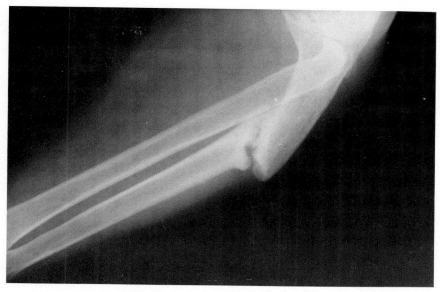

Fig. I.26. Nonunion of an oblique fracture of the junction of the proximal and middle third of the ulna. Note the sclerosis and covering over of the medullary canal.

X-ray examination reveals persistence of the fracture line, sclerosis and rounding off of the bone ends, and covering over of the ends of the medullary canals. There is no evidence of bone or callus bridging the defect (Fig. I.26).

Pseudoarthrosis

In nonunion, the bone ends are usually connected by dense fibrous or fibrocartilaginous tissue. In some instances, however, a false joint may form between the two fracture fragments. This joint is surrounded by a bursal sac containing synovial fluid and is called a pseudoarthrosis (Fig. I.27).

Malunion

Malunion occurs when there is union of the fracture with angulatory or rotary deformity (Fig. I.28).

Avascular Necrosis (Aseptic Necrosis)

Avascular necrosis occurs when the blood supply to a bone or a segment of bone has been interrupted. Initially following such insult, radiographically the bony architecture remains unchanged, but after a period of time the involved area becomes relatively more dense than the surrounding bones.

Nonunion and avascular necrosis are not necessarily coincident (Fig. I.29). Union of a fracture can take place despite avascular necrosis, or

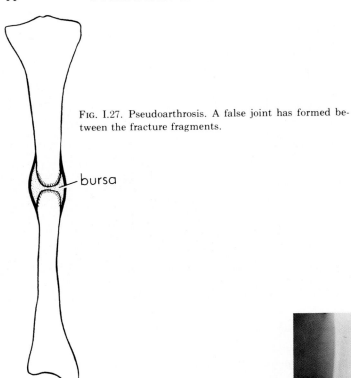

FIG. I.27. Pseudoarthrosis. A false joint has formed between the fracture fragments.

bursa

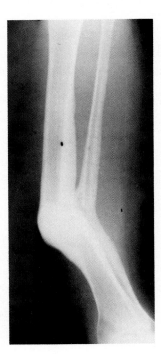

FIG. I.28. Malunion. A healed fracture of the junction of the middle and distal third of the tibia and fibula with lateral (valgus) angular deformity of the distal fragment or medial angulation of the fracture.

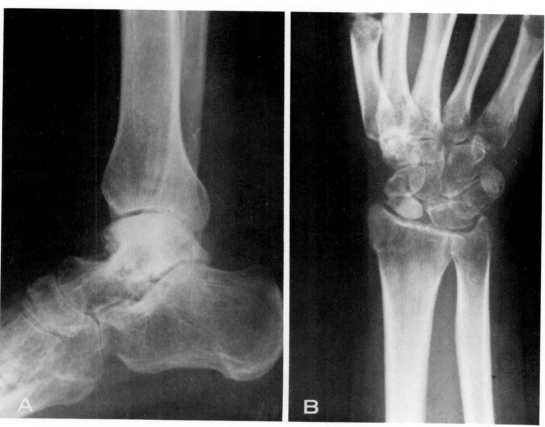

Fig. I.29.

(A) Avascular necrosis of the body of the talus. Note that the involved area is relatively more dense than the surrounding bones, and the fracture has united.

(B) Avascular necrosis and nonunion of the carpal navicular. Note that the proximal fragment is more dense and union has not occurred.

fracture fragments may remain viable despite the presence of nonunion. Thus four situations may arise: (1) complete union with both the proximal and distal portions remaining viable, (2) aseptic necrosis with union of the fracture, (3) nonunion of the fracture and viable bony fragments, and (4) nonunion of the fracture and aseptic necrosis.

FRACTURES IN CHILDREN

Fractures in children present special problems as there are certain features which are exclusively reserved for those fractures occurring in youthful bones.

These features include:

1. The presence of epiphyses, which in children are a frequent site of injury; as a consequence of the injury there may be growth disturbance.
2. The presence of epiphyseal lines, dense growth lines, secondary centers of ossification, and large nutrient foramina, all of which may be confused with fracture lines.
3. Incomplete fractures which commonly occur in children's bones because of their resilience or elasticity.
4. Rapid healing and great ability to remodel following fracture.

Because of the difficulties in diagnosis of injuries occurring in children's bones, it is imperative to obtain comparative x-rays of the opposite extremity to assist in diagnosis.

Anatomy

The Epiphysis

The epiphysis is that part of a bone which develops as a separate center of ossification, and is separated from the shaft by a layer of cartilage during the growing phase of the bone. Epiphyses are of several varieties, some of which are located at the ends of long bones and enter into the formation of a joint, while others occur at or near the ends of bones but do not enter into articulations. The presence of the epiphyses and the epiphyseal plates indicate that growth potential is still present, as once they have disappeared, growth in length ceases. Epiphyses are related to endochondral ossification, and several features should be understood. First, the epiphysis itself is not just the ossific nucleus that is visualized on x-ray but consists of the entire preformed cartilage region at the end of the bone, and thus the epiphysis is present before the ossific nucleus appears. Second, it is only when the center of ossification is present that a radiographic density appears. The cartilaginous epiphysis is not visualized because of the radiolucency of cartilage. At this point, frequently it is overlooked that the ossific density visualized on x-ray is only a portion of a much larger structure consisting of cartilage. Thus when interpreting radiographs of epiphyseal injuries, one should attempt to visualize the epiphysis as a whole and not just concentrate upon the ossified nucleus.

Another important point to be made is that the epiphyseal plate acts as the active growth area in relation to the length of the bone and not the epiphysis. The enlargement of the epiphysis itself is derived from the cartilage cells about the periphery of the epiphysis.

Essentially there are three types of epiphyses:

1. Pressure epiphysis.
2. Traction epiphysis.
3. Atavistic epiphysis.

Pressure Epiphyses. Pressure epiphyses are those epiphyses which are located at the ends of long bones and whose opposing surfaces will serve as the articulation for joints (Fig. I.30). The epiphyseal plates of pressure epiphyses contribute to the longitudinal growth of long bones. As previously noted, it is a common misconception that the epiphysis itself contributes to the growth of a long bone when, in fact, it is the epiphyseal plate that contributes to the longitudinal growth.

Traction Epiphyses. These epiphyses are nonarticular centers of ossification and serve as the attachments for tendons and ligaments. They may be found at the greater and lesser trochanters of the femur, the tuberosities and epicondyles of the humerus, and other sites. Growth of the epiphyseal plate of traction epiphyses may contribute to the shape of the bone, for example, the angulation of the femoral neck and shaft; however, they do not contribute to the length of the bone (Fig. I.30).

Atavistic Epiphyses. These epiphyses were phylogenetically independent bones and now have been incorporated onto another bone. An example is the coracoid process of the scapula, which is phylogenetically a separate bone and not part of the scapula.

Epiphyseal Injuries

Fractures of the epiphyses are one of the most common types of bone injury in childhood. Pressure and traction epiphyses are subject to different types of injury.

The cartilaginous epiphyseal line is potentially a zone of weakness, especially during periods of accelerated growth, and will tend to separate first, when subjected to injury, as opposed to rupture of ligaments or fractures of the adjacent bone. As fractures through the epiphyseal plate are at times difficult to recognize, comparative x-rays of the opposite extremity should be obtained.

Injuries to Pressure Epiphyses

Pressure epiphyses are subject to both shearing and compression type of forces, and tend to reproduce a common pattern of injury. Epiphyseal injuries produced by shearing stresses tend to cause displace-

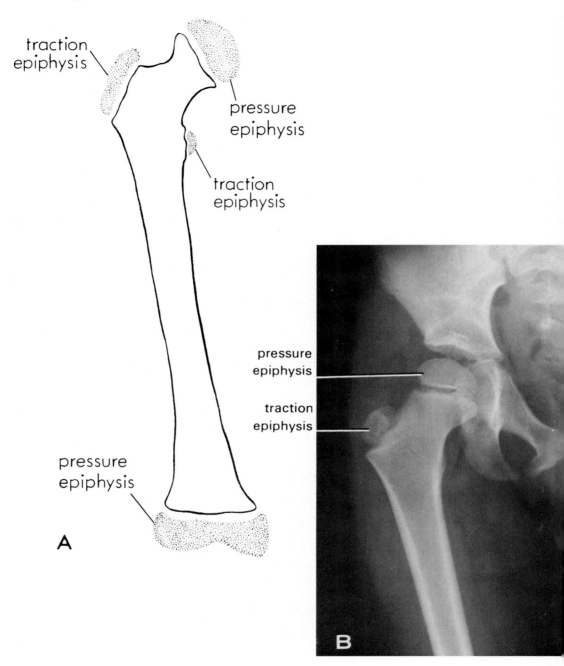

Fig. I.30.
    (A) Diagram of the femur demonstrating pressure and traction epiphyses.
    (B) Proximal femur demonstrating the above epiphyses.

ment of the epiphysis itself or to cause a small triangular bone fragment to be broken off from the adjacent metaphysis and accompany the displaced epiphysis. In compression injuries, the epiphysis itself may be split vertically, with the fracture line ending at the epiphyseal plate or continuing through the metaphysis. Compression forces may also produce crush injuries to the epiphyseal plate (Fig. I.31).

This pattern of injury has been classified by several experts in the past. Two of the most commonly used classifications are those of Aitken and of Salter and Harris. The Aitken classification has three types, as opposed to the Salter-Harris classification of five.

Salter-Harris Classification (Fig. I.31).

Type I. A Type I epiphyseal separation occurs when the fracture extends through the epiphyseal plate, resulting in displacement of the epiphysis.

Type II. In this injury, the direction of the fracture is similar to the Type I injury; however, a triangular segment of metaphysis is fractured and accompanies the separated epiphyseal fragment.

Type III. In a Type III epiphyseal fracture, the fracture line extends from the joint through the epiphysis to the epiphyseal plate, and then along the plate, dislodging a segment of epiphysis.

Type IV. In the Type IV injury, the fracture line passes from the joint surface, through the epiphysis, the epiphyseal plate, and the adjacent metaphysis.

Type V. This variety of epiphyseal injury results from a crushing type of force applied to the epiphysis, and the epiphyseal plate is injured.

In most epiphyseal injuries of the Salter-Harris Types I and II variety, growth is usually not affected; however, in Types III, IV, and V, growth considerations must be anticipated and the prognosis must be guarded.

Aitken Classification. In the classification proposed by Aitken, three types are described. Type I is a separation of the epiphysis with a small beak of metaphysis going with it; a Type II injury is splitting of the epiphysis up to the area of the epiphyseal plate, and a Type III variety is one in which the fracture line extends through the epiphysis and through the metaphysis.

Epiphyseal injuries may be described without referral to eponyms by simply describing the location of the separation; the direction of displacement of the epiphysis; the presence, direction, and location of any associated fracture; and the angulation occurring secondary to injury (Fig. I.32).

Injuries to Traction Epiphyses

Injuries to traction epiphyses are usually of an avulsion type. Again, the cartilaginous zone being a point of weakness, the epiphysis is pulled

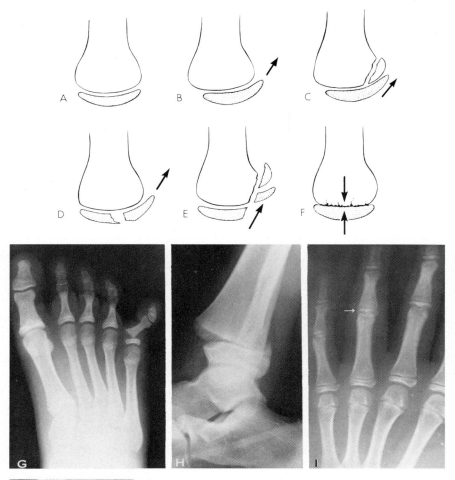

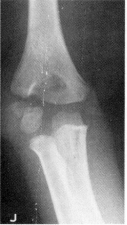

Fig. I.31. Types of injuries to pressure epiphyses (Salter-Harris classification).

(A) Normal epiphysis.

(B) Type I—Displacement of only the epiphysis.

(C) Type II—Displacement of the epiphysis associated with a fracture of the metaphysis.

(D) Type III—Fracture through the epiphysis to the epiphyseal plate.

(E) Type IV—Fracture through the epiphysis and metaphysis.

(F) Type V—Crush injury to the epiphyseal plate.

(G–J) Injuries to pressure epiphyses, Types I–IV.

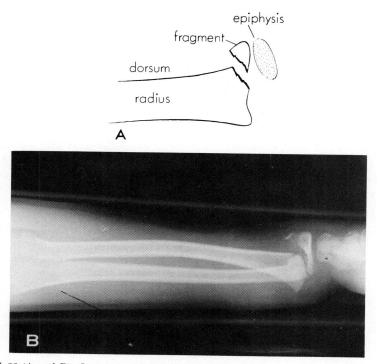

FIG. I.32 (A and B). Separation of the distal radial epiphysis with a fracture of the metaphysis and dorsal displacement of the distal fragment.

off by the violent contraction of the muscles, ligaments, and tendons which are inserted into it.

Examples of traction epiphyses subject to injury are: avulsion of the medial epicondyle at the elbow, the greater and lesser trochanters in the area of the hip, and the anterior superior and inferior iliac spines as well as the ischiotuberosities of the pelvis (Fig. I.33).

As the injuries to the traction epiphyses are usually avulsions, they may readily be described as avulsion fractures of the particular anatomical structure involved.

Incomplete Fractures

Because of the resiliency and elasticity of the bones of children, incomplete fractures of the long bones occur. There are two very common types of incomplete fractures in children which have special names: greenstick fracture and torus fracture.

Greenstick Fracture

This is an incomplete, angulated fracture producing bowing of the bone. It derives its name from it resemblance to a young branch which, when broken, breaks on its outer surface but is maintained intact on its inner surface, as compared to an old branch which breaks throughout its entirety. It should be noted that the broken cortex is always on the convex aspect (Fig. I.34).

Torus Fracture

In contrast to a greenstick fracture, a torus fracture is an incomplete fracture with a buckling of the cortex. Torus fractures are usually the

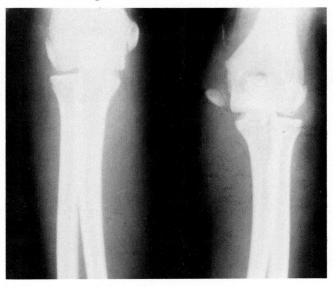

Fig. I.33. Avulsion fracture of the medial epicondyle, right elbow; comparative view of left elbow shows the normal anatomy.

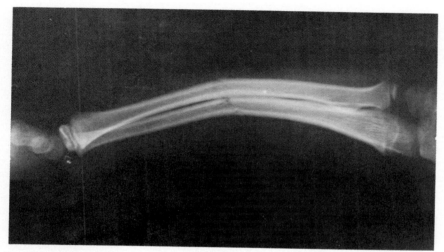

FIG. I.34. Greenstick fracture of the midshaft of both bones of the forearm.

result of compression forces and may be considered a type of compression fracture or, in fact, impaction fracture (Fig. I.35).

Remodeling

Another important consideration in children's fractures is remodeling (Fig. I.36). With continued epiphyseal growth, the distorted bony architecture may be corrected and varying degrees of angular deformity may ultimately result in a perfectly straight bone. Rotary deformity, however, cannot be remodeled. One may evaluate how much angular deformity will be spontaneously corrected through the use of a general rule which states that (1) the younger the child, (2) the closer the fracture is to the end of the long bone, and (3) if the displacement is in the direction of the plane of motion of the joint, the greater will be the remodeling. Thus greater angulation may be accepted in younger children if fractures occur toward the end of the bone with the angulation occurring in the direction of joint motion.

Review

The unique features of children's fractures have been covered, describing epiphyseal injuries, incomplete fractures, and remodeling. General fractures in children in other areas may be described in similar fashion to those of adult bones, as to direction, location, angulation, comminution, and whether they are open or closed.

For review, identify the fractures shown in the radiographs (Figs. I.I–I.L). The correct identification is given on page 385.

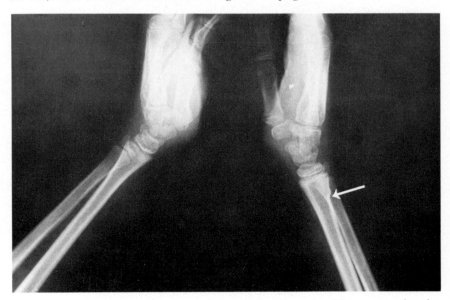

Fig. I.35. Torus fracture of the distal third of the radius on the right; comparative view of normal radius on the left.

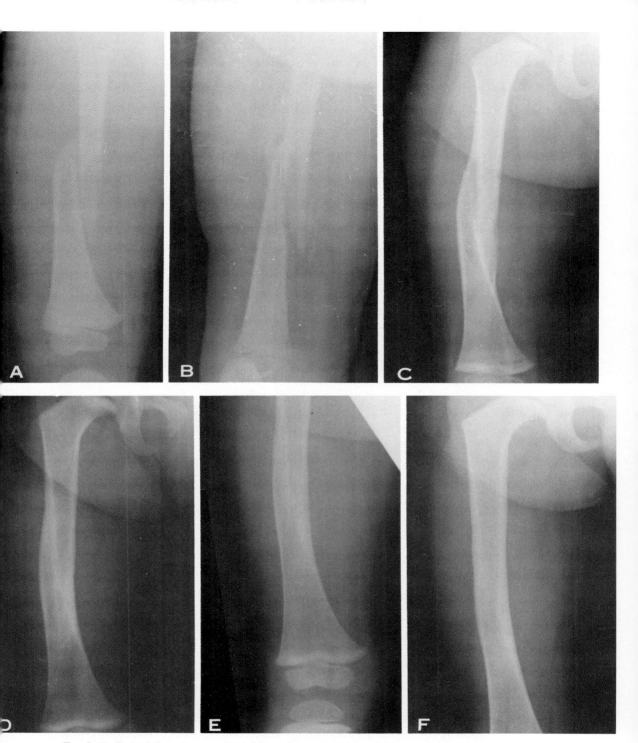

Fig. I.36. Remodeling of a complete oblique fracture of the midshaft of a femur in a 2-year-old child.

(A) Initial fracture.

(B) Periosteal new bone formation a few weeks after injury.

(C) Union of the fracture with primary callus 2 months post injury.

(D) Early remodeling and resorption of the primary callus.

(E) Further remodeling.

(F) At 13 months post fracture, note there is reestablishment of the medullary canal and continued remodeling almost restoring the normal architecture.

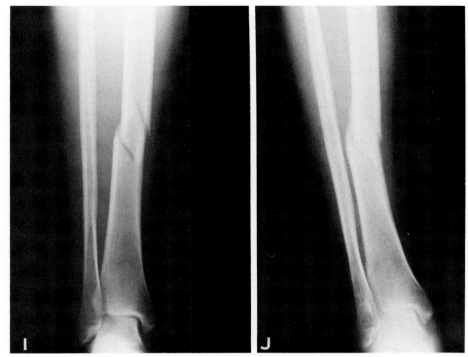

FIG. I.I   FIG. I.J

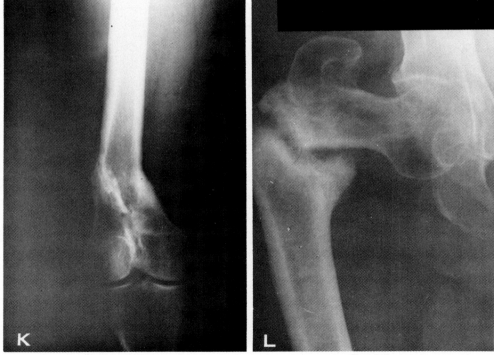

FIG. I.K   FIG. I.L

It should again be stressed that obtaining comparative x-rays on all injuries in children is imperative, as often the diagnosis is obscure without such diagnostic aid.

INJURIES TO JOINTS

Disruptions of joint architecture, as in the case with injuries to bones, lend themselves to ready identification through the use of the basic terminology hitherto presented.

Again, location of reference points, direction of disrupted parts, and associated injuries permit accurate description of joint dislocations as will be noted in the following section.

Anatomy

A joint or articulation expresses the relation of two or more bones to one another at their junction. Depending upon the location and the structural details of the articulation, this junction may be immovable, slighly movable, or freely movable. The composition of the linkage may be fibrous, cartilaginous, bony, or synovial in nature. Joints which have little or no motion have a fibrous, cartilaginous, or bony linkage, whereas those that are freely movable have articular cartilage overlying the opposing bone ends and a synovial lining.

Immovable Joints

Immovable joints are articulations which have no motion. These, for example, occur in the skull, where bony bridging occurs across the suture lines after closure.

Several terms describe the composition of the linkage which make up immovable joints (Fig. I.37).

Synchondrosis is a cartilaginous junction where the articulation is maintained by cartilage. This is usually a temporary state and occurs in the region of the growing ends of long bones between the epiphysis and the shaft. This residual cartilage may persist unossified for many years. Thus, an example of synchondrosis is the epiphyseal plate.

Synostosis is the bridging of a joint, or two bones by bony linkage. Synostoses occur through obliteration of a synchondrosis by bone as with closure of epiphyses, or of skull suture lines. It also may occur following fracture of two adjacent bones where cross bony bridging may connect the two bones (Fig. I.38).

Slightly Movable Joints

Slightly movable joints are joints which have very little motion and are usually bound together by fibrous tissue. The terms used to describe the linkage of these joints are syndesmoses or symphyses.

A *syndesmosis* (Fig. I.39A) is a joint held together by strong fibrous

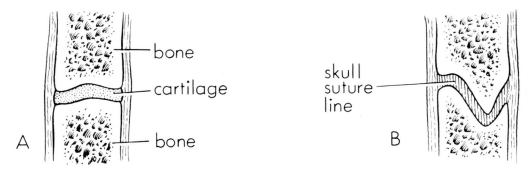

Fig. I.37. Immovable joints.
(A) Synchondrosis.
(B) Skull sutures which will close by bony bridging.

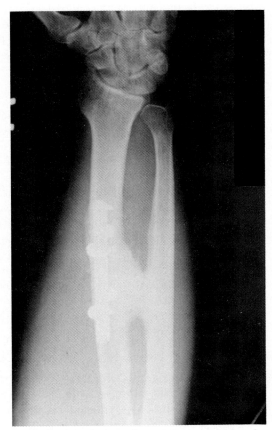

Fig. I.38. Synostosis secondary to cross bridging by bone following a fracture of both bones of the forearm.

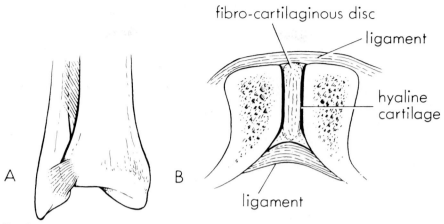

FIG. I.39.
(A) Syndesmosis (distal tibiofibular joint).
(B) Symphysis.

tissue which is well organized. Syndemosis may occur in the form of an interosseous membrane as between the radius and ulna, and tibia and fibula, or at the junction of two bones as at the distal articulation between the tibia and fibula, commonly referred to as the distal tibiofibular syndesmosis.

A *symphysis* (Fig. I.39B) is a joint where the opposing bony surfaces are covered with hyaline cartilage, are united by a fibrocartilaginous disc, and are stablizied by ligaments. Symphyses occur in the pubis and between the bodies of the vertebrae in the vertebral column.

Freely Movable Joints or Synovial Joints

The joints of the extremities which allow for more free movement are mainly synovial joints. Here, the opposing ends of the bones are covered by hyaline cartilage, stabilized by a joint capsule, and have a synovial membrane lining the inside of the capsule (Fig. I.40). The external appearance of an extremity shows that there is a variety of differently shaped joints. These varying shapes allow for varying degrees and directions of motion. Thus classification of synovial joints may be made based on the direction and the amount of motion that they allow.

Synovial Joint Classification:

1. *Plane or gliding joints.* Here the motion is a gliding or sliding movement and the opposed bony surfaces are relatively flat. This type of motion is found in the carpus, the tarsus, or the carpal metacarpal, or tarsal metatarsal joints.
2. *Uniaxial joints.* In uniaxial joints, motion is permitted in one plane (Fig. I.41).
   A. *Hinge or ginglymus joint.* This is a joint that allows motion

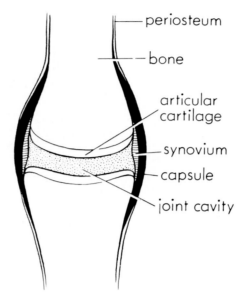

FIG. I.40. Synovial joint.

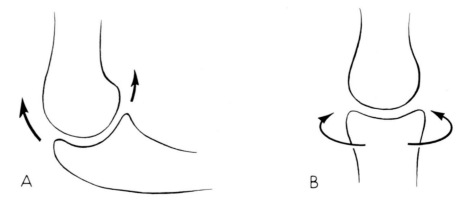

FIG. I.41. Uniaxial joints permit motion in one plane.
   (A) Ginglymus (hinge) joint—motion is at right angles to the long axis of the bone.
   (B) Trochoidal or pivot joint—motion is in the plane of the long axis of the bone.

at right angles to the long axis of the bone as in flexion and extension. An example of this is the ulnarhumeral articulation.

B. *Pivot or trochoidal joint*. This is also a uniaxial joint allowing motion about a single axis; however, in these joints the plane of motion is parallel to the longitudinal axis of the bone. This motion is seen at the radiohumeral articulation.

3. *Biaxial joints*. In a biaxial joint, motion is allowed in two directions at right angles to one another. Biaxial joints are either condyloid or ellipsoidal in shape. In a *condyloid joint*, one bony surface is a ball and the other a socket, whereas in an *elliposidal joint*, one surface is an oval and the other a socket. Examples of these joints are the metacarpophalangeal joints where the motion allowed is flexion, extension, abduction, and adduction.

4. *Multiaxial joints*. These joints allow for the greatest degree of motion of all. *Saddle joints*, such as the carpal metacarpal joint of the thumb allows for flexion, extension, abduction, and adduction, but, in addition, circumduction is possible. In *ball and socket joints* movement is permitted in an infinite number of directions, allowing motion in almost any plane. Examples of the ball and socket joints are the hip and the shoulder.

Classification of Joint Injuries

Dislocations and subluxations occur when there are structural alterations in the region of contact of the bones to one another. These alterations may be the result of congenital anomalies or acquired problems, the latter of which occur with injury; imbalance of muscle pull as in cerebral palsy, polio, or meningomyelocele; or changes in the contour of the articular surfaces of the bone secondary to diseases such as rheumatoid arthritis or osteoarthritis.

Dislocation

A dislocation is a complete disruption of the joint with loss of contact between the articulating surfaces of adjacent bones (Fig. I.42A).

Subluxation

A subluxation is a partial loss of continuity between the two opposing articular surfaces with some part of the opposing articular surfaces remaining in contact. Subluxations may be very mild to very severe where the joint is almost dislocated (Fig. I.42B).

Diastasis

A diastasis is a separation of normally joined parts, most commonly applied to slightly movable joints. Diastases occur in the region of the pubic symphysis or the distal tibiofibular syndesmosis (Fig. I.43).

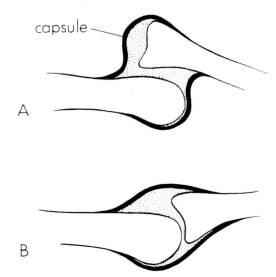

FIG. I.42.

    (A) Dislocation. Note that there is complete loss of contact of apposing articular surfaces.

    (B) Subluxation. Note that there is partial contact of the apposing articular surfaces.

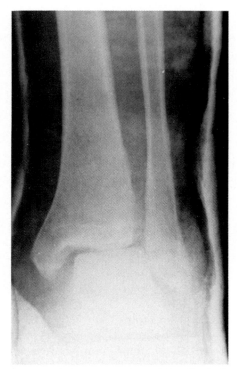

FIG. I.43. Diastasis. Note that there is separation of the distal tibia and fibula, leading to a widened ankle mortise.

Open Dislocation

As with fractures, subluxations, dislocations, or fracture dislocations may be of an open or compound nature. This occurs when the violence is severe enough to cause a soft tissue defect exposing the joint and the articulating bones to the outside environment. These injuries are referred to as open or compound dislocations, subluxations, or fracture dislocations. In these situations, because of the possibility of infection, the same *emergent consideration must be made as in open fractures*.

A *closed dislocation* is one in which the skin and soft tissues remain intact over the dislodged joint.

Establishing Location of Joint Injuries

Dislocations and subluxations are usually described by the joint involved; for example, dislocation of the hip, metacarpophalangeal joint, or shoulder (Fig. I.44A). In specific instances where the articulation is formed by more than two bones, there is variation in the terminology. In this situation, if disturbance of the articulation involves the two major bones comprising the joint, the dislocation is named for the joint involved. If the lesser bone of the three bone articulation is dislodged, then the dislocation or subluxation is described by the name of the bone displaced. This occurs, for example, in the region of the knee where there is an articulation of the femur, tibia, and patella. Dislocation of the tibia on the femur is designated as a dislocation of the knee; whereas if the patella is dislodged, it is referred to as a patella dislocation (Fig. I.44B) (see "Dislocation of Knee and Patella," page 112).

In areas such as the wrist where a group of bones can be dislocated as a unit or singly, the injury is described by the major joint involved or the individual bone displaced.

These latter situations will be further discussed in the section on specific location of injuries.

Direction of Dislocations

After establishing the location of the joint disrupted by the injury, we can proceed to describe the direction of the dislocation. In a two bone articulation or with disruption of the major components of a three bone articulation, the direction of joint disruption is assessed by describing the relation of the resting position of the distally placed bone to the proximal one, and dislocations are described as anterior, posterior, lateral, medial, superior, or inferior (Fig. I.45).

If the dislocation involves a single bone of a multiple bone articulation, as at the wrist, the relation of the resting position of this bone to the normal joint architecture is employed in its description. In a situation where the lesser bone of a three bone articulation is dislodged, the dislocation is described by the relation of the resting position of this bone

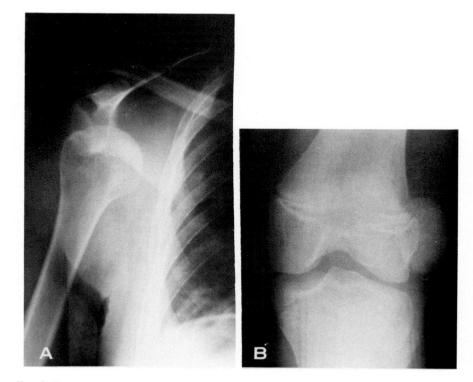

Fig. I.44.
  (A) Dislocation of the shoulder.
  (B) Dislocation of the patella. In an articulation consisting of three bones, dislocation of the lesser bone is named for the bone dislodged.

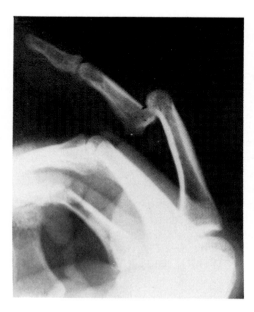

Fig. I.45. Volar dislocation of the middle phalanx of the index finger.

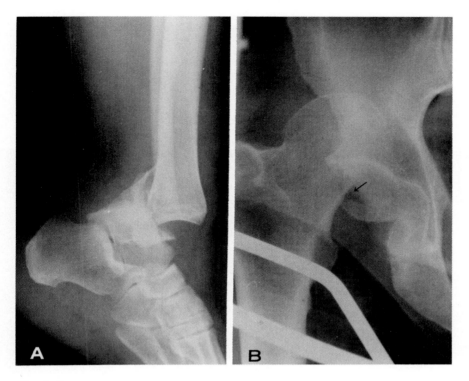

Fig. I.46.
(A) Posterior fracture dislocation of the ankle with fracture of the tibia and fibula.
(B) Fracture dislocation of the hip with fracture of the acetabulum.

to the rest of the joint. (Note Fig. I.44B in which there is a lateral dislocation of the patella.) Further consideration of the direction of dislocations will be made in the section on specific fractures.

Fracture Dislocation

Often at the time of injury, a fracture of one or both of the articulating bones may accompany the subluxation or dislocation. If this is present, it is considered to be a fracture dislocation and is described for the joint disrupted, the direction of the dislocation, and for the bone or bones involved in the fracture (Fig. I.46).

We may now pause to reflect on the vocabulary and our building of terms.

In review, subluxations or dislocations of joints are simply described by the name of the joint disrupted or bone dislodged, the location of the distal bone in relation to the proximal one, the presence of associated fractures and the nature of the injury, be it open or closed. Identify the fractures shown in the radiographs (Figs. I.M. and I.N.). Correct identification is given on page 385.

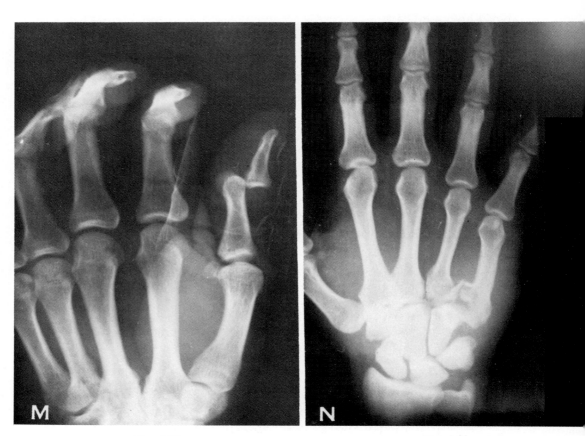

FIG. I.M   FIG. I.N

PART TWO

APPLICATION OF VOCABULARY TO SPECIFIC REGIONS

In Part II we can now apply the basic vocabulary to specific fractures and locations, and note the facility with which this terminology enables us to describe accurately the extent and nature of the pathology encountered.

HIP

ANATOMY

The hip joint is a synovial joint of ball and socket type and consists of the articulation of the head of the femur in a cuplike acetabulum (Fig. II.1). The head of the femur forms two-thirds of a sphere and is covered by an articular cartilage which ends at the junction of the head with the neck.

The neck of the femur is a pyramidal shaped section of bone which connects the head with the shaft in the region of the trochanters, and in so doing forms an angle with the shaft of approximately 135° in the anterior posterior plane, and a forward angle of approximately 15° when viewed from above, the latter referred to as anteversion (Fig. II.2). The inferior aspect of the neck is reinforced by a buttress of bone called the calcar femorale.

At the junction of the neck of the femur with the shaft, there are two protuberances, the greater and lesser trochanters. The *greater trochanter* is a large cancellous bony prominence at the upper outer end of the shaft of the femur which can be easily palpated through the skin. The *lesser trochanter* is a conical prominence projecting medially at the junction of the inferior aspect of the neck and the shaft of the femur.

On the anterior surface, the trochanters are joined by a rough, oblique ridge of bone called the intertrochanteric line which runs from the greater trochanter to a point just anterior to the lesser trochanter, and, on the posterior aspect, they are connected by a very prominent rounded ridge of bone called the intertrochanteric crest. The trochanters serve for the attachment of powerful muscles, the hip abductors (gluteus medius and minimus), inserting into the greater trochanter and the hip flexor, the iliopsoas, inserting into the lesser trochanter.

The articular capsule of the hip joint takes origin from the rim of the acetabulum and passes distally to insert anteriorly, the superficial fibers passing to the intertrochanteric line of the femur and the deep fibers to the base of the neck. Posteriorly, the fibers of the capsule wind

69

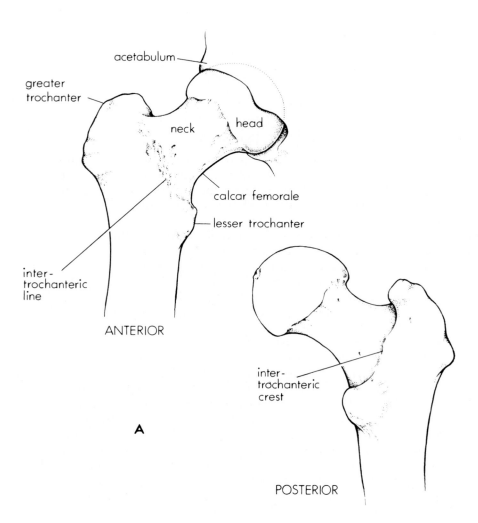

FIG. II.1. Bony anatomy of the hip joint.
(A) Anterior and posterior views of the proximal femur and acetabulum.

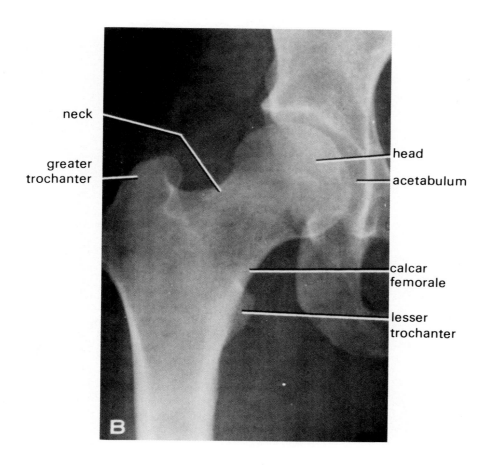

neck

greater
trochanter

head

acetabulum

calcar
femorale

lesser
trochanter

B

(B) Anteroposterior radiograph.

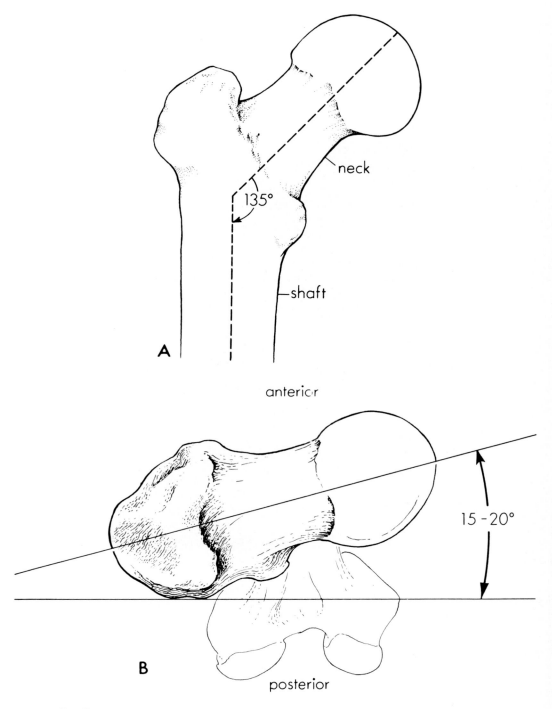

anterior

posterior

Fig. II.2.
(A) In the anterioposterior view (frontal plane) the normal neck shaft angle of the proximal femur is approximately 135°.
(B) Viewed from above, there is a forward angle of approximately 15°, referred to as anteversion.

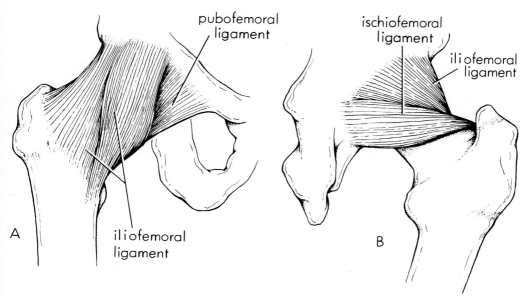

FIG. II.3. (A and B). The capsule of the hip joint extends anteriorly from the acetabulum to the intertrochanteric line and the base of the neck. Posteriorly, the capsule arises from the acetabulum and spirals anteriorly, covering only the proximal two-thirds of the neck of the femur. Three accessory ligaments, the iliofemoral, pubofemoral, and ischiofemoral ligaments, reinforce the capsule.

downward and forward in a spiral course, enveloping the head and the proximal two-thirds of the neck of the femur en route to their insertion anteriorly. A small synovial pouch protrudes from the margin of the fibrous capsule posteriorly and serves as a bursa for the obturator externus tendon. Thus posteriorly, the distal one-third of the neck is not covered by the joint capsule. Three accessory ligaments, the iliofemoral ligament anteriorly, the pubofemoral ligament inferiorly, and the ischiofemoral ligament posteriorly reinforce the capsule (Fig. II.3).

Within the capsule, the hip joint is lined by a synovial membrane except where there is articular cartilage. This synovial membrane is raised into several longitudinal loose folds around the neck of the femur called the retinaculum, in which the arteries ascend to supply the head of the femur.

The arterial blood supply to the femoral head is derived from several sources, with the major contribution coming from the lateral epiphyseal vessels which are branches of the medial femoral circumflex artery. These vessels enter the hip joint at the base of the femoral neck predominantly on the posterosuperior aspect, and travel along the femoral neck in the retinacular lining, closely apposed to the bone reaching and piercing the head at the junction of the head and neck. In addition to the lateral epiphyseal vessels, there are two other sources of blood supply to the head of the femur, (1) the artery of the ligamentum teres which variably contributes 10-30% of the total, and (2) the intramedullary blood vessels which travel from the femoral neck after the epiphysis has closed.

The clinical relevance of this blood supply is its extreme vulnerability to disruption in femoral neck fractures, dislocations of the hip, or by pressure phenomena in tense joint effusions leading to avascular necrosis of the femoral head.

Since the capsule attaches anteriorly to the base of the neck and the intertrochanteric line, the hip lends itself to division into three segments, namely an intracapsular region which contains the head and neck of the femur, an intertrochanteric region, and a subtrochanteric region. This division affords us a working vocabulary for the naming and description of hip fractures (Fig. II.4).

FRACTURES OF THE HIP

Fractures of the hip usually refer to those involving the proximal femur, including the head, neck, and trochanteric regions. Fractures of the acetabulum are usually considered as pelvic fractures.

FRACTURE NOMENCLATURE

In the preceding paragraphs, we have established reference points based on anatomical structure. Fractures occurring within these boundaries can now be classified (Fig. II.5):

   A. *Intracapsular fractures*. Fractures which occur within the confines of the capsule, namely those of the head and neck of the femur, are called intracapsular fractures. Because of the complexity of fractures in this region, further subclassification will be discussed subsequently.

   B. *Intertrochanteric fractures*. The intertrochanteric region is that section of bone just distal to the junction of the neck with the shaft, lying between the greater and lesser trochanters. Fractures occurring through the level of the trochanters are referred to as intertrochanteric fractures.

   C. *Subtrochanteric fractures*. Fractures occurring just beneath the trochanters are referred to as subtrochanteric fractures.

The division of the proximal femur into anatomic areas is more than just of academic interest, as fractures occurring in each of these locations have their own specific problems as to treatment, healing, and complications. In addition, surgical procedures and other hip pathology

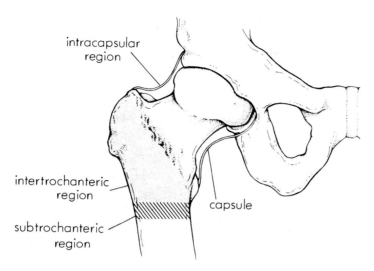

intracapsular
region

intertrochanteric
region

subtrochanteric
region

capsule

FIG. II.4. The anatomic structure of the proximal femur allows for division into three segments, an intracapsular region, an intertrochanteric region, and a subtrochanteric region.

can be described through these terms, for example, a subtrochanteric osteotomy, or a bone cyst in the intertrochanteric region.

Intracapsular Fractures

Intracapsular fractures are fraught with more complications than any of the other types of hip fractures, and thus require special attention. Further subclassification is necessary for the intracapsular area, and again this can be done by dividing the area into thirds, namely the subcapital area, the transcervical area, and the base of neck or basi-cervical area.

Subcapital fractures occur just distal to the articular margin of the head of the femur, whereas those passing through the neck are referred to as transcervical fractures. Fractures occurring at the junction of the neck and the shaft are referred to as base of neck (basicervical) fractures (Fig. II.6).

The complications of intracapsular fractures encountered most frequently are: (a) nonunion of the fracture, and/or (b) aseptic necrosis of the head of the femur, which results from interruption of its blood supply, and will be discussed shortly (see page 86). It should be noted that the more proximal the fracture, that is those closest to the head of the femur, the greater the incidence of complications.

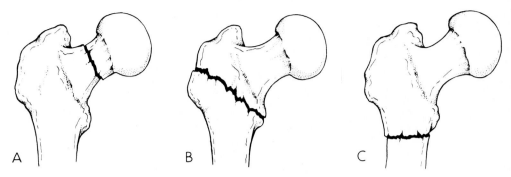

F<small>IG</small>. II.5. Fractures of the hip are described by the location in which they occur. Diagrammatically (A–C) Radiographs (D–F).

  (A) Transverse intracapsular fracture.
  (B) Oblique intertrochanteric fracture.
  (C) Transverse subtrochanteric fracture.

Thus hip fractures can readily be described by their anatomical location, initially being concerned with the intra- or extracapsular location, and then, if necessary, by further division of the intracapsular component.

Direction of Hip Fractures

The direction of hip fractures can be described, using our general terms as transverse, oblique, and comminuted, applied in routine fashion.

At one time emphasis was placed on the direction of hip fractures and its relation to fracture healing. In light of this, Pauwell established a classification in which intracapsular fractures were classified by their direction, noting the angle of the fracture line with the horizontal, as measured in the anterior posterior radiograph and basing this angular measurement on the postreduction x-rays. A Class 1 fracture formed an angle of 30° or less, a Class 2 fracture an angle of 30–70°, and a Class 3 fracture formed an angle of 70–90°.

His premise was that those fractures with a more horizontal fracture line would be subject to impacting forces with weight bearing and thus offer a better prognosis for healing than did more oblique fractures, which would be subjected to shearing forces (Fig. II.7). The Pauwell's classification is no longer commonly used but should be known by those interested in fractures.

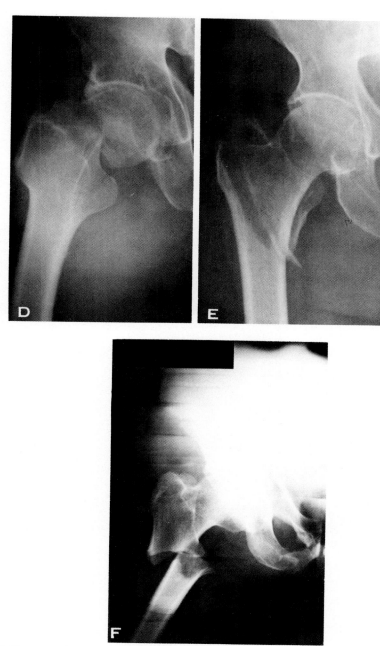

(D) Transverse intracapsular fracture.
(E) Oblique intertrochanteric fracture.
(F) Transverse subtrochanteric fracture.

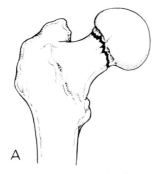
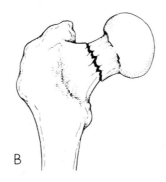
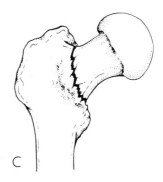

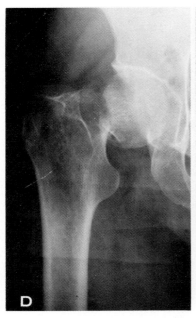
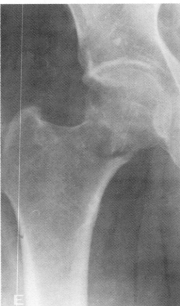
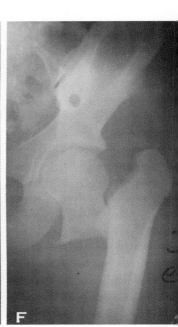

FIG. II.6. Subclassification of intracapsular fractures.
   (A) Subcapital fracture.
   (B) Transcervical fracture.
   (C) Base of neck fracture.
   (D) Transverse subcapital fracture.
   (E) Transcervical fracture.
   (F) Transverse fracture at the base of the neck.

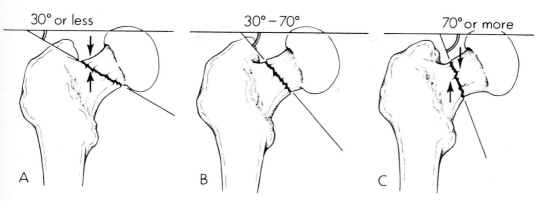

FIG. II.7. Pauwell's classification of hip fractures.

(A) Class I fracture. Note that the fracture line is somewhat horizontally directed, thus the forces of weight-bearing will theoretically produce a certain amount of impaction at the fracture site.

(B) Class II fracture.

(C) Class III fracture. In this injury the fracture line is more vertical, therefore, weight-bearing would effect a shearing force at the fracture surface.

Alteration of the Neck Shaft Angle

A factor, however, which is exceedingly important in fracture healing, especially of intracapsular fractures, is the status of impaction or distraction.

As previously stated, the normal neck shaft angle of the proximal femur is approximately 135°. Displaced fractures occurring in the region of the hip tend to alter this angle (Fig. II.8).

Coxa Valga

Coxa valga is any deformity of the hip occurring when there is an increase in the neck-shaft angle (Figs. II.8B and II.9). If at the time of fracture, the superior aspect of the neck of the femur is impaled into the head, the neck-shaft angle is increased and the fracture is considered to have assumed a valgus or abducted position.

Thus abduction or valgus fractures of the hip are those fractures which result in a neck-shaft angle greater than 135°. Since a state of impaction has occurred, the fracture has assumed a position of relative stability, and thus presents an excellent situation for fracture healing.

Coxa Vara

Coxa vara is a hip deformity occurring when there is a decrease in the normal neck-shaft angle to less than 135° (Fig. II.8C and II.10). If

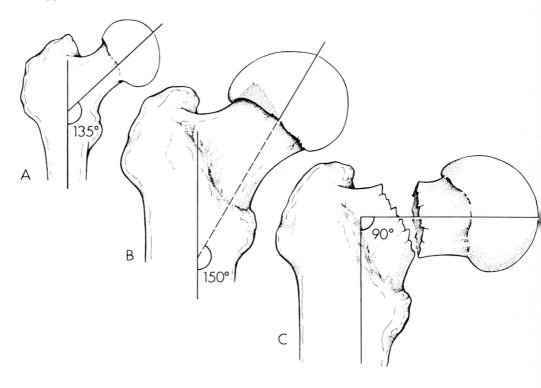

Fig. II.8.
   (A) Normal neck shaft angle of the proximal femur is approximately 135° in the antero-posterior plane.
   (B) Coxa valga. A valgus or abducted position occurs when the neck shaft angle formed is greater than 135°. Note that the fracture fragments are impacted.
   (C) Coxa vara. A varus or adducted position occurs when the neck shaft angle has become less than 135°. Note the distraction of the fracture fragments.

at the time of fracture, the neck-shaft angle becomes less than 135°, the hip is considered to be in varus or adduction. In contrast to the valgus fracture, this is a relatively poor situation for fracture healing as a status of displacement and distraction exists.

   The terms coxa valga or coxa vara are not reserved just for fractures, but may be applied to any situation when there is an alteration in the neck-shaft angle. This alteration may be congenital or acquired. Congenital coxa vara (Fig. II.11) occurs when the neck-shaft angle is less than 135° with no preexisting fracture. An acquired deformity may

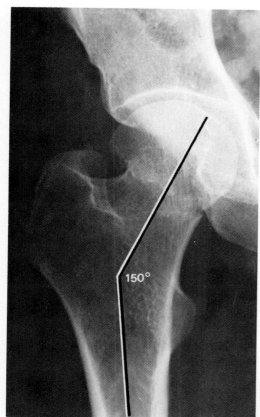

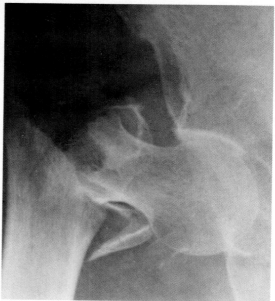

Fig. II.9. A transverse subcapital fracture in which the superior aspect of the neck has been impaled into the head assuming a valgus (abducted) position with the neck shaft angle greater than 135°.

Fig. II.10. Comminuted intertrochanteric fracture in a varus or adducted position.

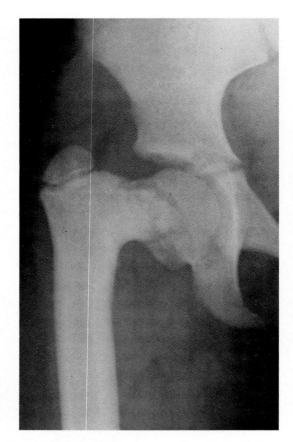

FIG. II.11. Congenital coxa vara. Although no fracture has occurred, the neck shaft angle is less than 135° and thus the hip is considered to be in varus. The epiphyses of the femoral head and greater trochanter are visible and may give the appearance of a fracture.

occur, for example, in association with poliomyelitis with paralysis of the lower extremity and involvement of the hip which often results in a coxa valga deformity.

FRACTURES OF THE GREATER AND LESSER TROCHANTERS

Direct Trauma

Fractures of the greater trochanter, at times, are the result of direct trauma. Fractures produced by this mechanism are usually comminuted, with little or no displacement. Separation and displacement of the greater trochanter is usually secondary to avulsion forces.

Fractures of the lesser trochanter almost never occur by direct trauma.

These fractures are described by the area involved with further application of our usual terminology.

Avulsion Forces

Avulsion fractures occur in the area of the greater and lesser trochanters, for these prominences serve for the attachment of strong ligaments and muscles. Separation of the greater trochanter usually occurs as the result of forceful muscular contraction by the abductors and external rotators of the hips, whereas the lesser trochanter is avulsed by the powerful iliopsoas muscle (Fig. II.12).

These fractures lend to application of our routine terms and are designated as avulsion fractures of the greater or lesser trochanter.

FRACTURE OF THE FEMORAL HEAD

Fractures of the femoral head are rare but do occur and are usually associated with dislocation of the hip. At the time of injury, a segment of the head is sheared off, the fragment of which is composed of articular cartilage, or articular cartilage and the underlying subchondral bone. These fractures, designated as fractures of the femoral head, may also be considered chondral or osteochondral fractures of the femoral head (Fig. II.13).

PATHOLOGIC FRACTURE OF THE HIP

The proximal femur is a common site for pathologic fractures. These fractures are usually the result of local disease, such as bone tumors or metastatic lesions, and, at times, are due to radiation therapy.

Pathologic fractures are usually located in the intertrochanteric or subtrochanteric regions, but at times are intracapsular in nature. The lesion is described by its location and the fact that it is pathologic must be noted (Fig. II.14).

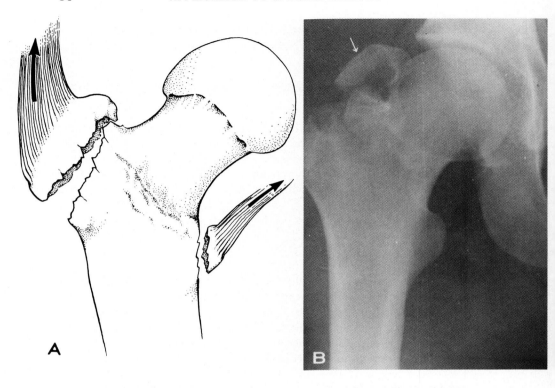

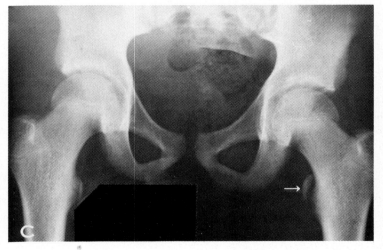

Fig. II.12.

(A) Avulsion fractures of the greater and lesser trochanters. Note the forces of muscle contraction which produce the avulsion and distraction.

(B) Avulsion fracture of the greater trochanter.

(C) Avulsion fracture of the epiphysis of the lesser trochanter on the right—the other extremity is included for comparison.

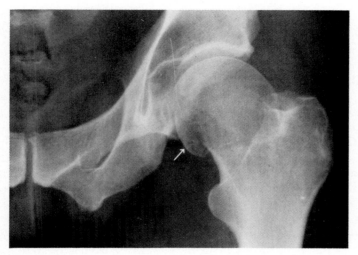

Fig. II.13. Fracture of the femoral head. Note the triangular fragment at the infero-medial aspect of the head of the femur.

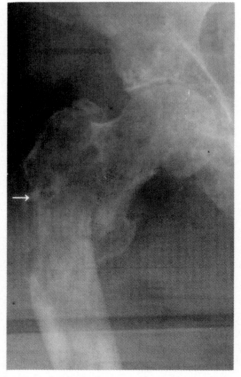

Fig. II.14. Pathologic subtrochanteric fracture. Note the mottled appearance of the diseased bone.

COMPLICATIONS OF HIP TRAUMA

Avascular Necrosis

Avascular necrosis of the femoral head develops when its blood supply is interrupted. There are multiple etiologies of avascular necrosis, such as prolonged use of cortisone, sickle cell anemia, Gaucher's disease, and alcoholism, to mention a few. When avascular necrosis is secondary to trauma, however, it results from interruption of the blood supply by a fracture occurring through the femoral neck, or rupture of the posterior capsule as can occur in a dislocation of the hip.

With avascular necrosis, radiographically, initially the bony architecture remains unchanged and thus the early roentgenographic pictures are normal. Later, the involved area becomes relatively more dense as compared to the adjacent bone (Fig. II.15). Subsequently the head of the femur can collapse and assume an irregular shape. These final stages result in joint incongruities and subsequent osteoarthritis of the hip. Consequently, studies must be continued over a period of many months to demonstrate the development of this pathology. Fracture healing may take place with union at the fracture site despite the presence of avascular necrosis.

Nonunion

Nonunion occurs as the result of an unsatisfactory reduction, inadequate immobilization, or, as with avascular necrosis, due to interruption of the blood supply to the head of the femur, secondary to trauma.

Nonunion is represented by the persistence of the fracture line and sclerosis of the fracture margins, without bony bridging (Fig. II.16). Nonunion may exist with or without the presence of avascular necrosis.

Other complications of hip trauma include osteoarthritis, malunion of fractures, myositis ossificans, and peripheral nerve injuries. The last usually occurs as a result of a posterior dislocation of the hip and most commonly involves the peroneal branch of the sciatic nerve.

FRACTURE OF THE HIP IN CHILDREN

Fractures of the hip may occur in children, secondary to trauma, and in general, can be classified, as previously described, by their location, (intracapsular, intertrochanteric, subtrochanteric), the direction of the fracture and the deformity, whether comminution exists, and if the underlying lesion is pathologic (Fig. II.17).

Specific situations, however, are present in children which are not present in adults. One of these is the presence of the *capital femoral epiphysis*.

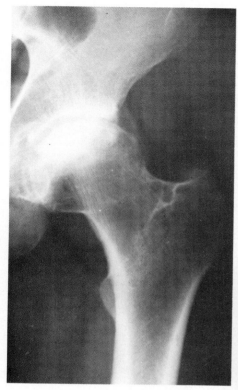

FIG. II.15. Avascular necrosis. Note the increased density of the superior medial aspect of the head of the femur.

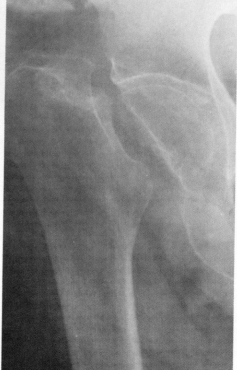

FIG. II.16. Nonunion secondary to a transverse subcapital fracture. Note that there is no increased density of the head of the femur, and thus no avascular necrosis is evident at this time.

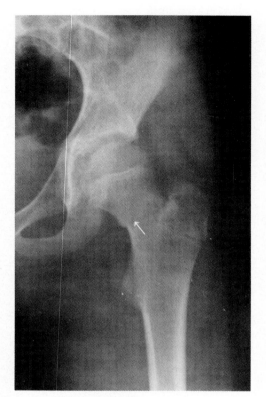

FIG. II.17. Transverse transcervical fracture in a child. Note the epiphyses of the greater trochanter and head of the femur which are not to be misinterpreted as fracture lines.

Slipped Capital Femoral Epiphysis

At the upper end of the femur in children, separation or slipping of the capital femoral epiphysis may occur. This condition usually occurs in children between the ages of 12 and 16 years when there is a period of rapid growth. The entity is referred to as slipped capital femoral epiphysis. Although no definite etiology has been established, a specific type of patient is usually predisposed to this abnormality, namely the Fröhlich type of obese, sexually underdeveloped male, or the slender rapidly growing individual. In the majority of cases, the slipping is gradual, usually occurring in an insidious fashion, with the head gradually being displaced inferiorly and posteriorly from the femoral neck. As a result of the inferior displacement of the head a varus deformity of the hip ensues; whereas, when the head is displaced posteriorly, the neck of the femur assumes an anteriorly displaced position. The combination of these deformities causes the shaft of the femur to assume a position of adduction and external rotation.

This displacement, however, may also take place following acute trauma. This occurrence, termed an "acute slip," is in reality a form of fracture displacement which can occur at other epiphyseal sites as well.

X-ray examinations of both the acute and chronic slips will reveal, in the anteroposterior projection, inferior displacement of the head of the femur, whereas the lateral view will reveal the posterior displacement of the femoral head. It should be noted, however, that the pathology may be visible on only one radiographic view, i.e., either the anteroposterior or the lateral.

Acute slips, however, should be differentiated from chronic or slowly progressing slips and this can be done radiographically. In the latter, there is gradual molding of the femoral neck, with callus formation being evident along the posteroinferior aspect of the femoral neck. Concomitantly, resorptive changes result in the formation of a rounded prominence at the anterosuperior margin of the femoral neck. Since these changes require considerable time to be manifested, the callus formation and remodeling will not be present in the acute slipped femoral capital epiphysis (Fig. II.18).

At times, an acute traumatic episode may produce an acute displacement (slip) of the femoral head on a chronically displacing head. In this situation there would be evidence of remodeling of the neck, indicating the site of the chronic displacement. However, this remodeling would not extend to the level of the acutely displaced capital epiphysis.

Avascular Necrosis

A second situation that complicates hip fractures in children is the high incidence of avascular necrosis of the head of the femur. This complication occurs following intracapsular fractures, as well as intertrochanteric fractures, and presents itself, as in adults, as a delayed radiographic and anatomic change (Fig. II.19).

Avulsion Fractures

Avulsion fractures of the greater and lesser trochanters in children are not uncommon. These areas represent traction epiphyses and, before fusion, present points of weakness more susceptible to avulsion fractures as a result of muscular violence (see Fig. II.12). Avulsion fractures may occur as an isolated injury or associated with dislocation of the hip in children. Traumatic dislocation of the hip in children, however, is rare. These injuries are named for the epiphysis involved.

DISLOCATION OF THE HIP

A dislocation of the hip occurs when the head of the femur is dislodged from the acetabulum. Dislocations of the hip may occur with or without associated fractures of either the head of the femur or the acetabulum.

The type of dislocation is designated by the final resting position of the femoral head in relation to the acetabulum.

Posterior Dislocation

Posterior dislocations of the hip are the most common type and are present if the head of the femur comes to rest posterior to the acetabulum (Figs. II.20A and II.21). On the anteroposterior x-ray, the head of the femur appears superior to the acetabulum. These injuries are designated as posterior dislocations of the hip.

Anterior Dislocations

An anterior dislocation is one in which the head of the femur is anterior to the acetabulum.

Anterior dislocations can be further subdivided into pubic and obturator or peroneal dislocations.

In pubic dislocations, the head of the femur lies over the pubic crest, whereas in an obturator dislocation the head of the femur reaches the obturator foramen (Figs. II.20 and II.22).

Central Dislocations

A central dislocation occurs when a force is transmitted through the head of the femur which fractures the lateral wall of the acetabulum and thrusts the femoral head into the pelvis (Fig. II.23). The force applied causing the fracture usually is directed against the greater trochanter.

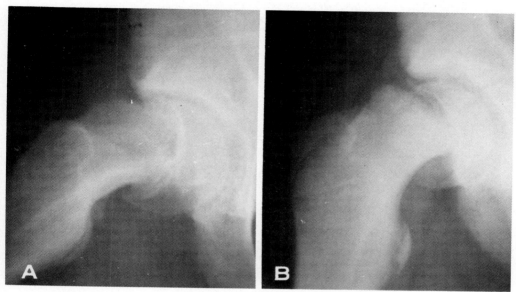

Fig. II.18.

(A) Chronic slip. In a chronic slip, there is reshaping of the superior aspect of the neck of the femur and a filling in at the inferior aspect of the neck near the head.

(B) Acute slip. In this entity, the posterior and inferior displacement of the head is present without remodeling and reshaping of the neck.

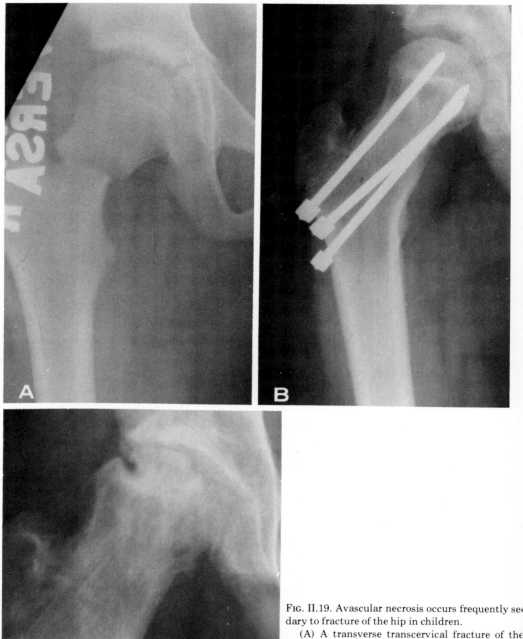

FIG. II.19. Avascular necrosis occurs frequently see dary to fracture of the hip in children.

(A) A transverse transcervical fracture of the mur has occurred.

(B) Open reduction and internal fixation was formed on the day of injury.

(C) Fourteen months post injury there is irr larity and increased density of the superior aspe the head of the femur, revealing the presence avascular necrosis. The pins have been removed the fracture is healed. These changes produce j incongruity and ultimately osteoarthritis of the hi

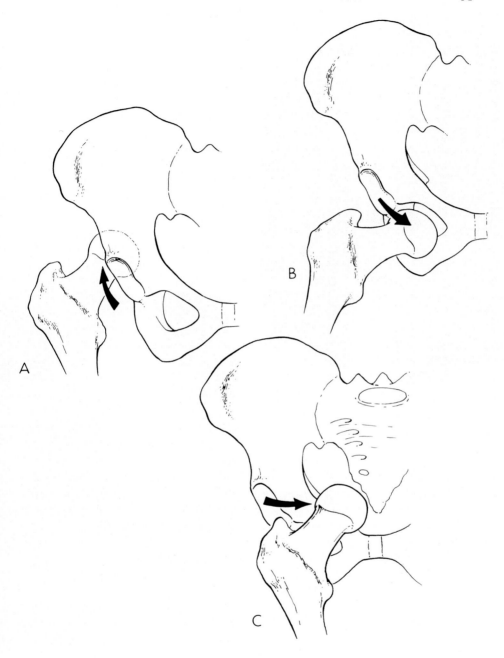

FIG. II.20. Dislocations of the hip are named by the final position of the head of the femur in relation to the acetabulum.

(A) Posterior dislocation. The head is posterior to the acetabulum and usually superior.

(B) Anterior (obturator dislocation). The head of the femur has come to rest in the area of the obturator foramen.

(C) Anterior (pubic dislocation). The head of the femur lies over the pubic crest.

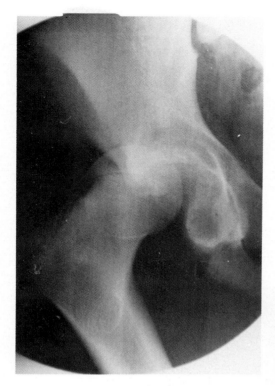

FIG. II.21. Traumatic posterior dislocation of the hip in a child.

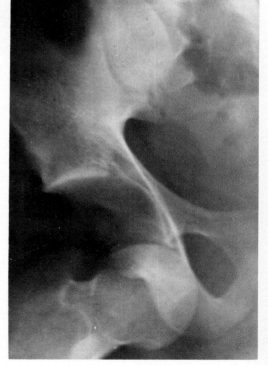

FIG. II.22. Anterior dislocation. Note that the head of the femur is inferior to the acetabulum, near the obturator foramen.

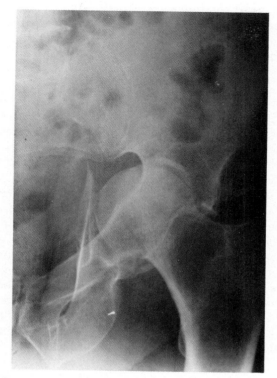

FIG. II.23. Central fracture dislocation of the hip. The head of the femur is displaced into the pelvis with fracture of the medial portion of the acetabulum.

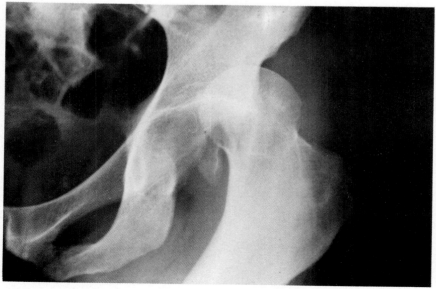

FIG. II.24. Fracture dislocation of the hip. A posterior dislocation of the hip with a fracture of the posterior rim of the acetabulum.

The result is marked comminution of the wall of the acetabulum with medial displacement of the head of the femur into the pelvis. These injuries, often classified as central dislocations of the hip, are, in fact, fracture dislocations and may be classified as such.

Dislocations and Associated Fractures

Dislocations of the hip are, at times, associated with marginal fractures of the acetabulum, the degree of severity and stability of the dislocation, following reduction, being proportional to the size of the acetabular fragment dislodged. This situation usually occurs with posterior dislocations which, in fact, shear off the posterior rim of the acetabulum (Fig. II.24).

Dislocation of the hip may also be associated with fractures of the femur, namely fracture of the femoral head, fracture of the femoral neck, separation of the upper femoral epiphysis, and fracture of the shaft of the femur.

Thus dislocations and fracture dislocations of the hip are named for (1) the position of the femoral head following the dislocation, either anterior or posterior and, if anterior, by its subclassification; (2) by the presence of an associated fracture either of the pelvis, acetabulum, or femoral head or shaft (for example, a posterior dislocation of the hip with a fracture of the posterior rim of the acetabulum); and (3) central dislocation where the head is driven into the pelvis.

Dislocations of the hip are orthopedic emergencies, as avascular necrosis of the head of the femur may be related to the length of time the hip is left unreduced. The magnitude of the trauma, however, may also play an important role in causing this complication.

Review

Identify the fractures illustrated (Figs. A–D). Correct identification is given on page 385.

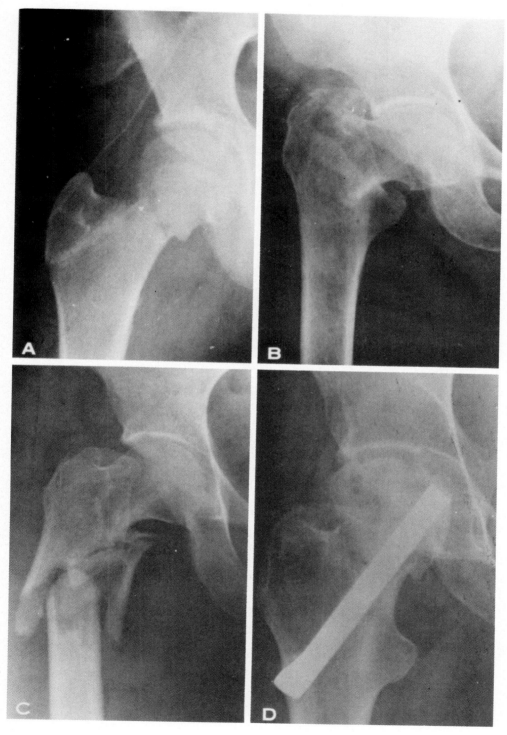

THE KNEE

ANATOMY

The knee joint is a synovial joint formed by the articulation of the distal femur, proximal tibia, and the posterior aspect of the patella. Two major articulations are present in the knee, the tibiofemoral articulation and the patello-femoral articulation, with division of the tibiofemoral joint into a lateral and medial compartment, produced by the intraarticular cruciate ligaments.

Distal Femur (Fig. II.25). The distal end of the femur is broadened by two large prominences, a larger medial and smaller lateral condyle. Bulging above and within the curvatures of the condyles are the femoral epicondyles which give origin to the collateral ligaments of the knee.

The femoral condyles are covered with cartilage in front, below, and behind. Posteriorly, the condyles of the femur blend together and, in so doing, form a U-shaped intercondylar notch. Anteriorly, the condyles meet, forming a V-shaped depression providing a groove in which the patella moves. The anterior surface of the femoral condyles articulates with the posterior surface of the patella, and the distal and posterior surfaces of the condyles articulate with the tibia.

Proximal Tibia (Fig. II.25). The proximal tibia is expanded in relation to the shaft. These lateral and medial enlargements are referred to as the lateral and medial condyles. The articular surfaces, called the tibial plateaus, are flattened, covered by articular cartilage, slightly concave in nature, and receive the condyles of the femur. Between the two plateaus is the raised, roughened intercondylar eminence which ends in two small prominences, the anterior and posterior tibial spines. The articular surfaces of the tibial plateaus are deepened by disclike menisci.

Anteriorly, distal to the tibial condyles, there is a bony prominence, the tibial tubercle, into which the ligamentum patellae inserts.

The proximal fibula does not enter into the knee joint articulation but serves for the attachment of supporting ligaments and muscles of the knee.

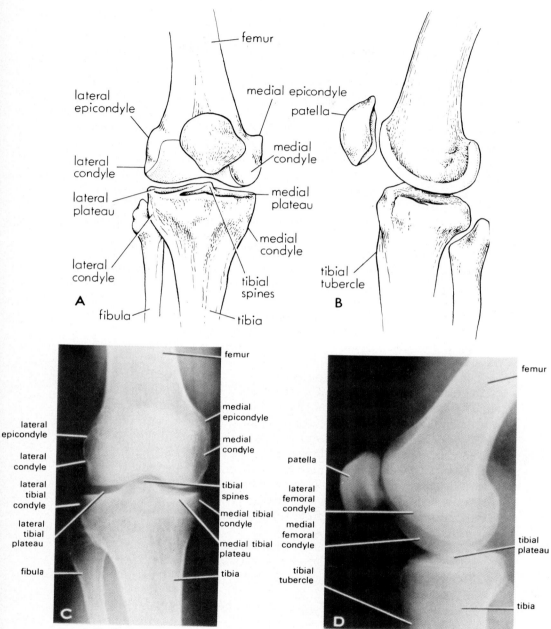

FIG. II.25. Bony anatomy of the knee.
(A) Anterior view.
(B) Lateral view.
(C) Anteroposterior radiograph of normal knee.
(D) Lateral projection of normal knee.

Patella. The patella is a large somewhat triangular sesamoid bone which develops in the tendon of the quadriceps muscles. It arises from a single center of ossification which appears at 2½ years of age in the female and 3 years of age in the male. As with all sesamoid bones, the patella has no periosteum. The posterior surface of the patella is covered by articular cartilage and, with flexion and extension of the knee, glides in the intercondylar groove of the femur. In this position, it produces a prominence in the course of the tendon of the quadriceps femoris and the patella tendon, which alters the direction of pull and improves the functional efficiency of the quadriceps mechanism (Fig. II.26).

Supporting Structures. If the knee joint was to depend solely on the bony architecture of the opposed ends of the femur and tibia, it would be a very unstable arrangement. Stability is obtained by the presence of strong collateral ligaments which are reinforced by aponeuroses and tendons, and a strong capsule and intraarticular ligaments (Fig. II.27).

The articular capsule of the knee arises from the femoral condyles and attaches below the tibial plateaus and the borders of the menisci. The capsule is reinforced and inseparable from the ligaments and aponeuroses apposed to it. Anteriorly, expansions from the quadriceps, fascia lata, and iliotibial band reinforce it by forming the medial and lateral patella retinacula, and laterally and medially it is reinforced by the collateral ligaments.

The collateral ligaments are two strong retaining structures on each side of the knee, attached not to the centers of the condyles but to the epicondyles of the femur. The tibial collateral ligament is a broad, flat band composed of two layers, a superficial and a deep, with the superficial layer extending from the epicondyle of the femur to the medial surface of the shaft of the tibia. The deep fibers of the tibial collateral ligament extend from the epicondyle of the femur to the medial condyle of the tibia, and the ligament is intimately bound to the articular capsule of the knee on the medial side. The fibular collateral ligament is a cordlike structure which extends from the lateral epicondyle of the femur to the head of the fibula.

The aponeurotic tendons of the quadriceps mechanism are attached to the margins of the patella, as the patella retinacula or expansion, and extend to the level of the attachment of the patella tendon at the tibial tubercle.

The cruciate ligaments lie within the confines of the joint, cross each other in the form of an X, and extend from the intercondylar surface of the femur into the intercondylar region of the tibia. The anterior cruciate ligament arises from the inner aspect of the lateral femoral condyle and passes to the front of the intercondylar eminence of the tibia.

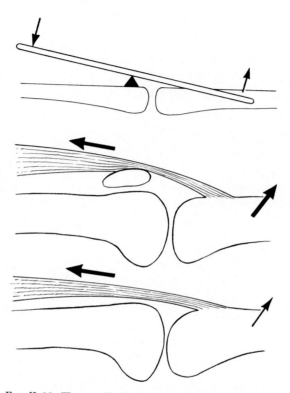

Fig. II.26. The patella forms a prominence in the tendon of the quadriceps muscle. This prominence provides a fulcrum which changes the direction of pull and improves the mechanics of the quadriceps mechanism.

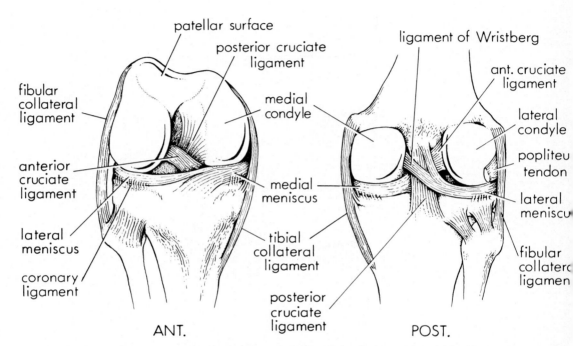

FIG. II.27. Anterior and posterior views of the supporting ligaments which provide stability to the knee.

The posterior cruciate ligament extends from the medial condyle of the femur and passes to an area posterior to the tibial spines.

The inner aspect of the capsule of the joint is lined by an extensive synovial membrane. The synovium reflects onto the bone (except where there is articular cartilage) and surrounds the cruciate ligaments, extends beneath the aponeuroses of the vasti, and reduplicates itself in the shape of fringelike folds.

Thus the anatomic architecture of the knee allows for the establishment of several reference points (Fig. II.28):

1. The femoral condyles.
2. The tibial plateaus.
3. The patella.
4. The tibiofemoral articulation.
5. The patellofemoral articulation.

This division affords us working landmarks for naming and describing fractures and dislocations about the knee.

INJURIES TO THE KNEE

Injuries to the knee may result from direct and indirect trauma and may affect the bony elements or the soft tissue structures.

Based on the previously described anatomy, we have established various reference points. We can now apply our general fracture terms to the structures in and about the knee.

Thus we can describe the injuries to the knee as those occurring at:

1. The distal femur.
2. The proximal tibia.
3. The patella.
4. The tibiofemoral articulation.
5. The patellofemoral articulation.

FRACTURE NOMENCLATURE

The more common fractures about the knee are the supracondylar fractures and intercondylar fractures of the femur, as well as depressed fractures of the tibial plateaus and fractures of the patella.

Distal Femur

Fractures of the distal femur are described in relation to the femoral condyles and can occur above and through the femoral condyles.

Supracondylar Fractures

Fractures occurring above the femoral condyles are referred to as supracondylar fractures (Fig. II.29). A more sophisticated description should include the direction of these fractures, and can be described in our usual terms as transverse, oblique, and comminuted. Because of the

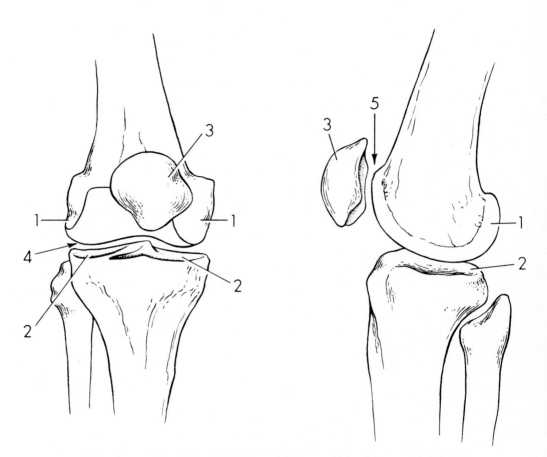

FIG. II.28. Division of the anatomic architecture of the knee into established reference points: (1) femoral condyles, (2) tibial plateaus, (3) patella, (4) tibiofemoral articulation, and (5) patello-femoral articulation.

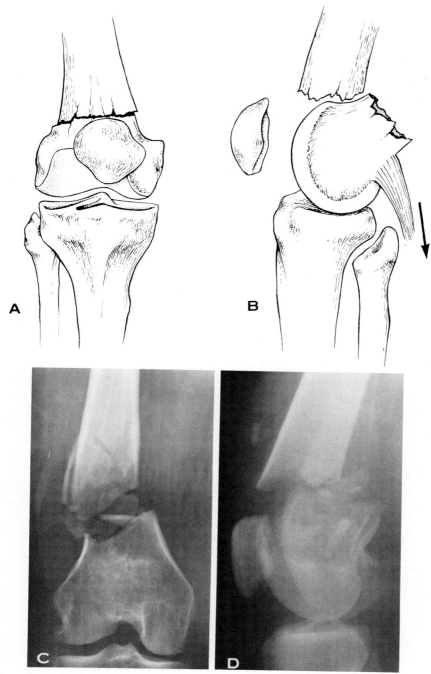

FIG. II.29. Supracondylar fractures.

(A and B) Diagrammatic representation of a transverse supracondylar fracture of the femur. Note the pull of the gastrocnemius muscle, causing the distal fragment to be rotated posteriorly.

(C and D) Anteroposterior and lateral radiograph of a comminuted supracondylar fracture of the femur.

pull of the gastrocnemius muscle on the distal fragment, these fractures are frequently angulated posteriorly.

Intercondylar Fractures

Fractures passing through the condyles are described as intercondylar and transcondylar fractures. Intercondylar fractures may occur in various patterns, depending on the direction and comminution of the fracture. Single fracture lines may be present and involve one or both condyles, in transverse, oblique, and more vertical patterns, and at times may extend into the joint. These fractures are described by noting the direction of the fracture and which condyle is involved. Transverse fractures extending through both condyles are referred to as transcondylar fractures (Fig. II.30). Comminuted intercondylar fractures may occur in many different directions and these may be described by the pattern formed by the fracture lines. The most common patterns are those of T- or Y-shaped fractures. These fractures usually extend into the knee joint and, therefore, are intraarticular (Fig. II.31).

Proximal Tibia

As the fractures of the articular aspects of the femur are described in relation to the femoral condyles, fractures of the proximal tibia are related to the tibial plateaus or adjacent areas.

Tibial Plateaus

The most common fracture of the proximal tibia is fracture of the plateau. Such fractures occur when a force is applied to either the lateral or medial aspect of the knee, resulting in a valgus or varus tilt and causing the hard femoral condyle to be driven into the softer tibial plateau. This stress causes a compression of the bone and a depression of the articular surface and subchondral bone of the tibia into the underlying cancellous bone. These fractures are, in fact, impaction fractures and are defined as depressed fractures of either the medial or lateral tibial plateau. Most commonly, the lateral plateau is involved (Fig. II.32). Frequently, as an associated injury with plateau fracture, there is rupture of the contralateral collateral ligaments; however, if significant depression occurs, instability of the knee results despite the fact that the retaining ligaments may still be intact. This occurs because the normal retaining buttress of the plateau no longer can support the femoral condyle (Fig. II.33).

The tibial plateaus may be involved by other fractures which are usually the result of indirect violence. Falls on the feet cause crushing injuries to the tibial plateaus and result in displaced or nondisplaced, longitudinal fractures, or Y- or T-shaped fractures as may occur in the femoral condyles (Fig. II.34).

Avulsion fractures involving the tibial plateaus also occur as the result

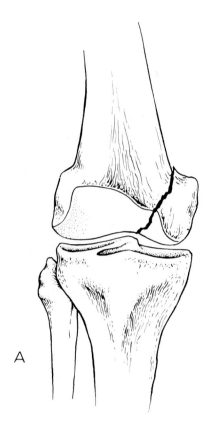

A

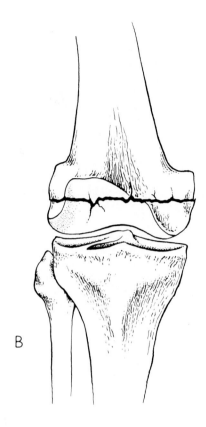

B

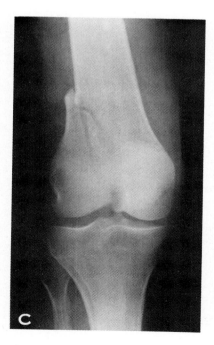

C

FIG. II.30. Intercondylar fractures.

(A) Oblique fracture of the medial femoral condyle.

(B) Transverse, transcondylar fracture of the femoral condyles.

(C) Oblique fracture of the lateral femoral condyle.

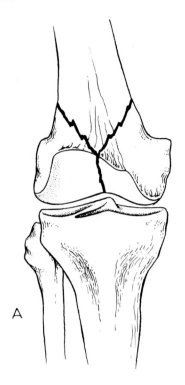

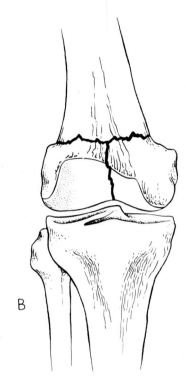

A

B

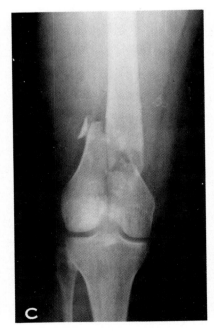

C

Fig. II.31

(A) Y-shaped intercondylar fracture of the distal femur.

(B) T-shaped intercondylar fracture of the distal femur.

(C) A Y-shaped intercondylar fracture of the distal femur. Note that in both the diagrams and radiograph the fracture extends into the joint and thus it is intraarticular in nature.

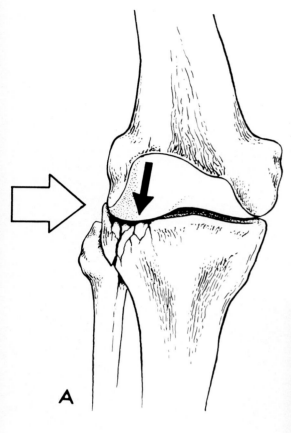

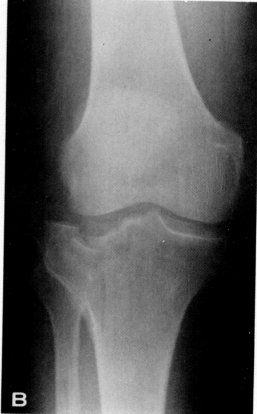

Fig. II.32.

(A) A valgus force applied to the knee causes the hard femoral condyle to be driven into the softer tibial plateau, resulting in depression of the tibial plateau.

(B) Depressed fracture of the lateral tibial plateau. Note the depression of the articular surface and sub-chondral bone into the underlying cancellous bone.

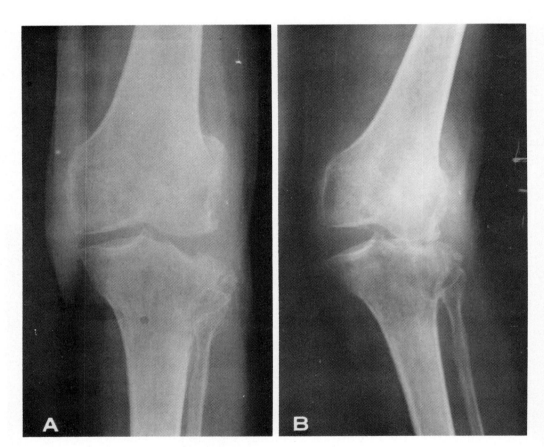

Fig. II.33.
(A) Depressed fracture of the lateral tibial plateau.
(B) Instability of the knee to valgus stress caused by the lack of the normal supporting buttress of the plateau of the femoral condyle is revealed.

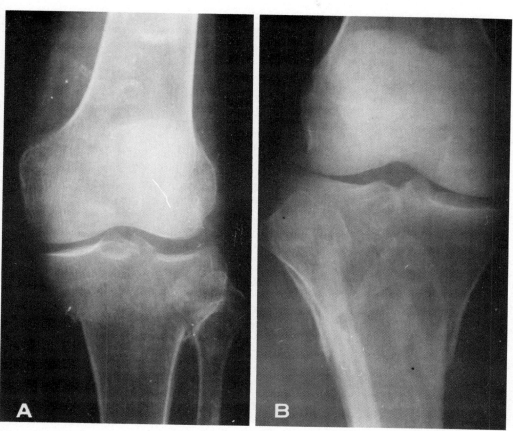

FIG. II.34.

(A) Comminuted V-shaped fracture of the tibial plateaus with a slight depression of the lateral tibial plateau. (Note that the V is inverted.)

(B) Comminuted Y-shaped fracture (inverted Y) of the tibial condyles.

of abduction or adduction trauma to the knee. These injuries are classified as avulsion fractures of the plateau involved (see "Avulsion Fractures").

Patella

The patella, because of its superficial position, and location within the substance of the quadriceps tendon which subject it to the forces of the quadriceps muscle, is susceptible to fractures from both direct or indirect trauma. Fractures of the patella are described by the direction of the fracture (which are usually transverse, comminuted, or stellate in nature), the area of the patella involved, and the amount of displacement (Fig. II.35). In complete fractures which divide the bone in a horizontal pattern, distraction of the fracture fragments usually occurs despite the mechanism of injury because of the pull of the quadriceps mechanism.

Avulsion Fractures

As previously described in the section of anatomy, the knee joint is supported by many strong ligaments and tendons. Avulsion injuries occur and are caused by abduction and adduction stresses applied to the leg, as well as forceful flexion, extension, and rotary injuries. As avulsion fractures affect areas where strong ligaments and tendons insert, the regions of the femoral epicondyles, the rim of the tibial plateaus, the tibial condyles, the anterior and posterior tibial spines, the tibial tubercle, and the patella are predisposed.

These avulsion fractures are described in routine manner, applying basic vocabulary to the anatomic area involved. They may also be referred to, if indicated, as intraarticular fractures and, by virtue of the mechanism of injury, are usually displaced (Fig. II.36).

Tibiofemoral and Patellofemoral Articulations

Disturbances of the tibiofemoral articulation and patellofemoral articulation are primarily concerned with dislocations and fracture dislocations, and will be discussed together. Dislocations about the knee can occur at either the tibiofemoral articulation or the patellofemoral articulation.

Dislocation of the Knee

As previously stated, articulations of more than two bones have a variation in terminology.

A dislocation of the knee principally refers to disruption of the tibiofemoral articulation, whereas disruption of the patellofemoral articulation is referred to as a dislocation of the patella.

Dislocations of the knee occur when there is disruption of the ligaments and loss of contact of the apposing articular surfaces of the tibia and the femur. The dislocation is described by the final resting position

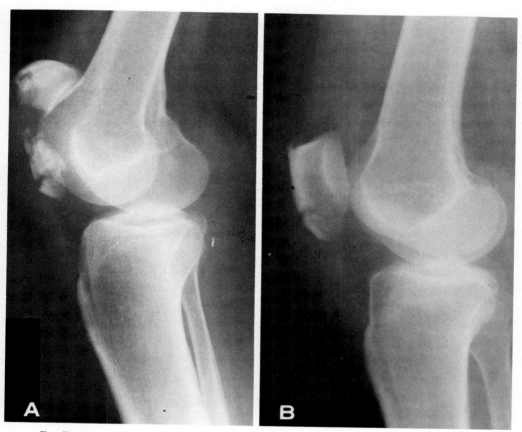

FIG. II.35.

(A) Transverse fracture of the patella with distraction, and comminution of the distal fragment.

(B) Nondisplaced transverse fracture of the distal third of the patella.

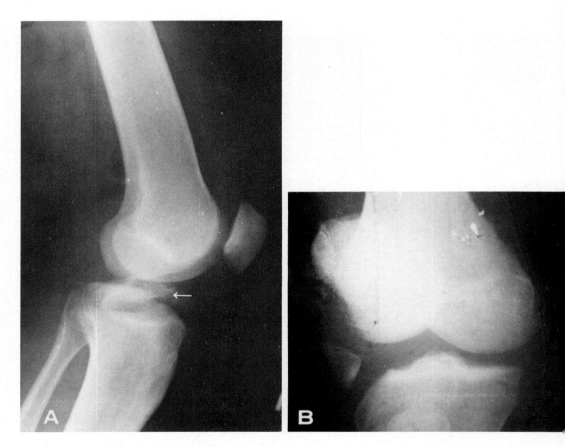

FIG. II.36. Avulsion fractures.
  (A) Avulsion fracture of the tibial spine.
  (B) Avulsion fracture of the lateral tibial plateau. Note involvement of the articular surface, and that the fragment is rotated 90°.

of the tibia in relation to the femur. An anterior dislocation is one in which the tibia is anterior to the femur, whereas a posterior dislocation occurs when the tibia is posterior to the femoral condyles. Lateral and medial dislocations can also occur (Fig. II.37).

Dislocation of the Patella

Disruption of the patellofemoral articulation results in a dislocation of the patella, with the patella being displaced from the intercondylar groove. The patella is almost always displaced laterally, and the dislocation is described by the final resting position of the patella in relation to the distal femur (Fig. II.38).

Fracture Dislocations

Frequently fractures may accompany dislocations of the knee or the patella. For example, with a lateral dislocation of the patella, a fracture of the lateral femoral condyle may occur. In like fashion with dislocations of the knee, fractures of the tibial plateaus or femoral condyles may accompany the dislocations. These injuries are referred to as fracture dislocations and are described by the joint involved, the direction of the dislocation, and the bone fractured.

Injuries of the Knee in Children

Epiphyseal Injuries

Fractures about the knee in children, prior to epiphyseal closure, may involve the distal femoral or the proximal tibial epiphyses.

Injury to the distal femoral epiphysis usually results in separation of the epiphysis through the epiphyseal plate and may be described by application of our basic vocabulary related to epiphyseal injuries (Fig. II.39).

Separation of the entire proximal tibial epiphysis is rare; however, avulsion of the anterior aspect of the tibial epiphysis occurs more frequently (Fig. II.40). These lesions may be described in routine fashion, noting the epiphysis involved, the direction of displacement, and the presence of associated fractures.

Other Injuries

In general, fractures and dislocations about the knee in children may be described in similar fashion to those of adult injuries.

Review

Identify the fractures illustrated (Figs. A-E). Correct identification is given on page 385.

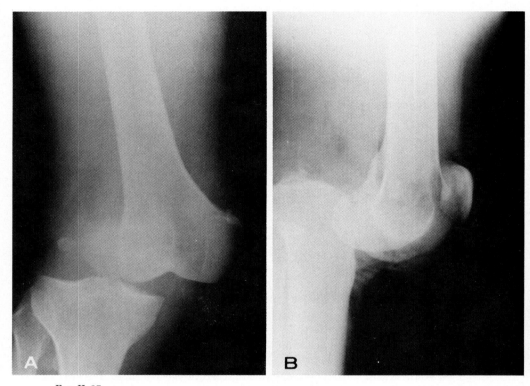

Fig. II.37.
   (A) Lateral dislocation of the knee and the patella. Note that the patella has remained in its normal position in relation to the tibia.
   (B) Posterior dislocation of the knee.

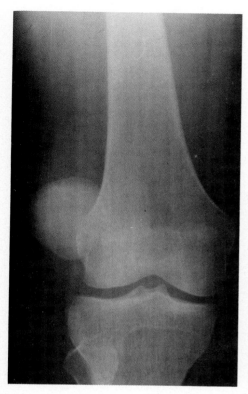

FIG. II. 38. Lateral dislocation of the patella. Note the
normal position of the tibiofemoral articulation.

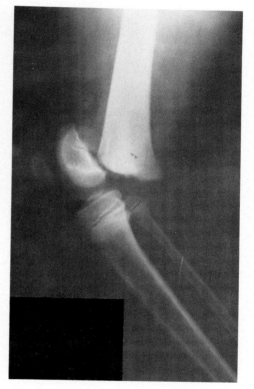

FIG. II. 39. Separation of the distal femoral epiphysis
with anterior displacement of the epiphyseal fragment.

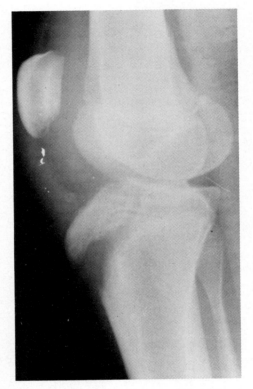

FIG. II.40. Avulsion of the anterior aspect of the proximal tibial epiphysis (tibial tubercle).

FIGS. A–D.

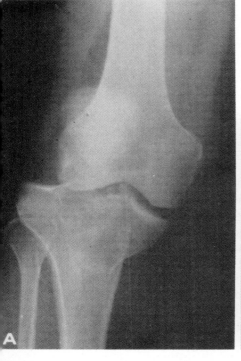

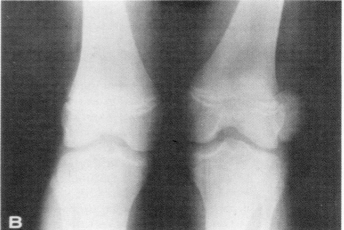

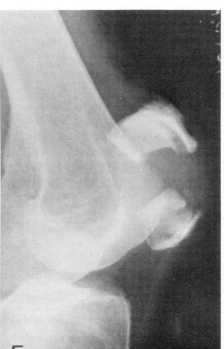

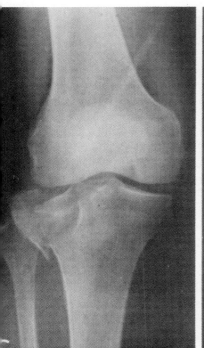

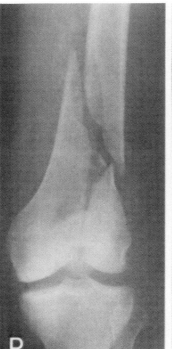

119

THE ANKLE

ANATOMY

The ankle is a synovial joint of the hinge or ginglymus variety, composed of an articulation of three bones: the distal end of the tibia, the distal end of the fibula, and the talus (Figs. II.41 and II.42).

The distal aspect of the tibia is somewhat broadened and includes an inferior articular surface which articulates with the superior surface of the body of the talus, a lateral surface with a triangular depression for the articulation with the fibula (the fibular notch), and a blunt projection which extends inferiorly as the most distal projection of the medial aspect of the tibia called the medial malleolus.

The lateral malleolus is the expanded, somewhat pointed distal end of the fibula which extends approximately one-half to three-quarters of an inch below the tip of the medial malleolus. Its medial aspect consists of an articular facet for the talus and a larger surface for its articulation with the tibia. The distal projecting ends of the tibia and fibula or malleoli, plus the inferior surface of the tibia, form an ankle mortise into which the dome-shaped talus fits. The inner aspects of both the lateral and medial malleoli and inferior margin of the distal tibia are covered with articular cartilage and articulate with the cartilage covered dome of the talus.

Just superior to the ankle mortise, there is a junction or articulation of the tibia and fibula, bound together by strong fibrous tissue ligaments called the distal tibiofibular syndesmosis. In this region, the fibula lies posterior and lateral to the tibia and thus, radiographically, on anterior-posterior projection, is overlapped by the tibia (Fig. II.42).

An interosseous membrane joins the lateral crest of the tibia and the medial crest of the fibula, and extends from below the superior tibiofibular joint distally to be continuous with the distal tibiofibular syndesmosis.

The architecture of the ankle affords bony stability which is further reinforced by the articular capsule and the collateral ligaments. The capsule surrounds the joint and is attached proximally to the margins of the tibia and fibula and below to the talus in front of and behind its superior articular surface.

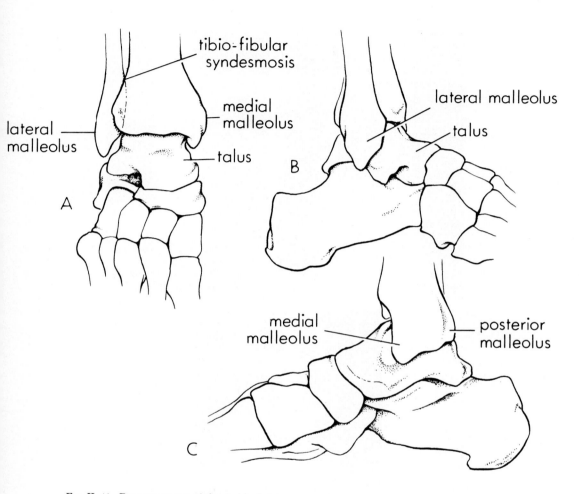

Fig. II.41. Bony anatomy of the Ankle Joint.
(A) Anterior view.
(B) Lateral view.
(C) Medial view.

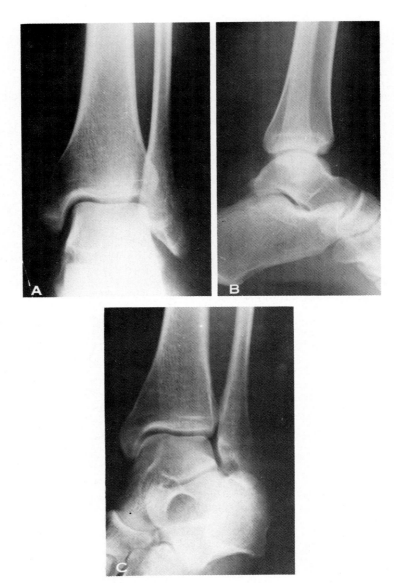

FIG. II.42. The normal ankle.

(A) On anteroposterior view, the distal fibula is not only lateral but also posterior to the tibia and thus there are overlapping shadows at the tibiofibular syndesmosis.

(B) Lateral view.

(C) Oblique view. Note that in the oblique view there is no overlap of the tibia and fibula. This view is designed to visualize the tibiofibular syndesmosis.

The collateral ligaments of the ankle joint are exceedingly strong and lie at the sides of the ankle, attached to and radiating down from the malleoli to insert into the tarsal bones (Fig. II.43). The medial collateral ligament (deltoid ligament) is a strong, somewhat triangular structure attached to the tip of the medial malleolus, and flares out inferiorly to insert into the talus, calcaneus, and navicular. It is composed of four components, named according to their attachments, the anterior talo-tibial ligament, the tibionavicular ligament, calcaneotibial ligament, and the posterior talotibial ligament. The lateral ligaments, the anterior one of which is so frequently injured in sprains of the ankle, are three in number. They attach to the tip of the lateral malleolus and insert into the talus and calcaneus. These are the anterior talofibular ligament, the calcaneofibular ligament, and the posteror talofibular ligament.

A synovial membrane lines the capsule, and extends upward between the apposed surfaces of the ends of the tibia and fibula, and well forward onto the neck of the talus.

Thus, by virtue of its anatomical structure, the ankle allows for ready division into components (Fig. II.44):

1. The medial and lateral malleoli.
2. The inferior articular aspect of the distal tibia.
3. The distal tibiofibular syndesmosis.
4. The ankle joint.

INJURIES OF THE ANKLE

Injuries to the ankle are common and are usually the result of abduction, adduction, internal and external rotation trauma which results in both shearing and avulsion type fractures, dislocations, and fracture dislocations.

Thus with the established anatomical reference points, injuries of the ankle may be described by applying our routine vocabulary based on location:

1. Fractures of the medial and lateral malleoli.
2. Articular fractures of the distal tibia.
3. Separation of the distal tibiofibular syndesmosis.
4. Dislocation or fracture dislocation of the ankle joint.

FRACTURE NOMENCLATURE

Fractures of the Malleoli

Medial and Lateral Malleoli

A fracture of the medial malleolus is one that involves the distal projection of the tibia, whereas that of the lateral malleolus involves the distal projection of the fibula (Fig. II.45).

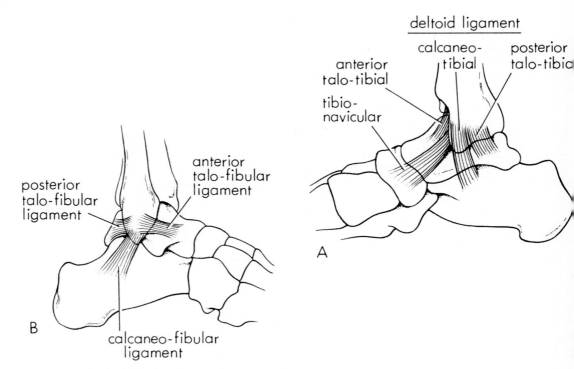

FIG. II.43. Collateral ligaments.
 (A) Medial collateral or deltoid ligament with its insertion into the talus, calcaneus, and navicular.
 (B) Components of the lateral collateral ligament.

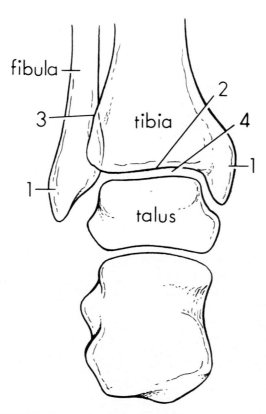

FIG. II.44. Anatomic structure of the ankle allows for classification of fractures by area: (1) malleoli, (2) inferior articular aspect of the distal tibia, (3) tibiofibular syndesmosis, and (4) ankle joint.

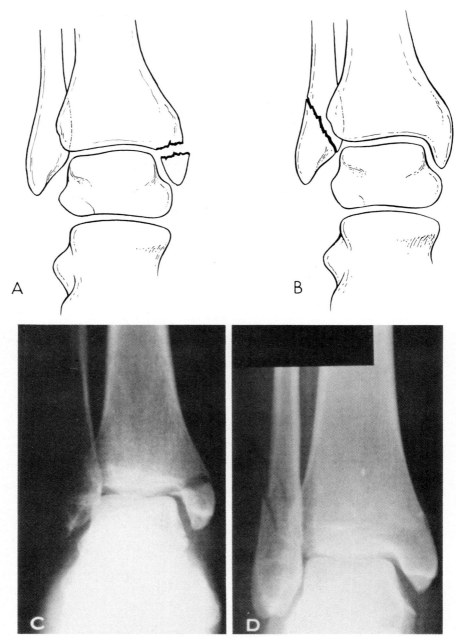

Fig. II.45. Fractures of the malleoli.
  (A) Diagrammatic representation of a transverse fracture of the medial malleolus.
  (B) Diagrammatic representation of an oblique fracture of the lateral malleolus.
  (C) A transverse fracture of the medial mallelous.
  (D) An oblique fracture of the lateral malleolus.

Fractures of the malleoli are caused by shearing and torsional stresses, produced by abduction, adduction, and rotary forces applied to the ankle. As the malleoli serve as the attachments for strong ligaments, these forces produce avulsion fractures when the ligaments are placed under tension, or a shearing fracture when the talus is forced against the involved malleoli (Fig. II.46). These injuries may occur alone or in conjunction with each other.

Fractures of the medial malleolus are intraarticular in nature and produce a disturbance of the ankle mortise, with or without displacement of the malleolar fragment. Lateral malleolar fractures need not be intraarticular as they can occur above the articular margin and produce a disturbance of the mortise only if the distal tibiofibular syndesmosis is ruptured (Fig. II.47).

Applying our basic terminology, fractures of the malleoli are named for their anatomical location (lateral or medial), the direction of the fracture or the presence of comminution and displacement, and the level of the fracture in relation to the inferior articular surface of the tibia. Avulsion fractures may be described as such.

Posterior Malleolus

The posterior articular aspect of the distal tibia is continuous with the medial malleolus and presents as a thickened buttress of bone which projects slightly distally. Although it is not truly a malleolus, fractures involving the articular surfaces of this area are referred to as posterior malleolar fractures (Fig. II.48).

Bimalleolar Fractures

If both the lateral and medial malleoli are fractured, the fracture is called bimalleolar. Any combination of bimalleolar fractures may exist as to direction, displacement, and comminution, for example, there may be an oblique fracture of the lateral malleolus with a transverse fracture of the medial malleolus, or a transverse fracture of the lateral malleolus with an oblique fracture of the medial malleolus (Fig. II.49).

Thus any time both malleoli are fractured, it is referred to as a bimalleolar fracture, with further elaboration using basic terminology, if desired.

Trimalleolar Fracture

If the medial and lateral malleoli, as well as the posterior articular margin of the tibia or posterior malleolus are fractured at the same time, this is designated a trimalleolar fracture (Fig. II.50).

Articular Fracture of the Distal Tibia

Intraarticular fractures of the distal tibia can occur when a severe upward force is applied by the talus through the distal tibia as may occur with a fall from a height. The intraarticular fracture of the tibia pro-

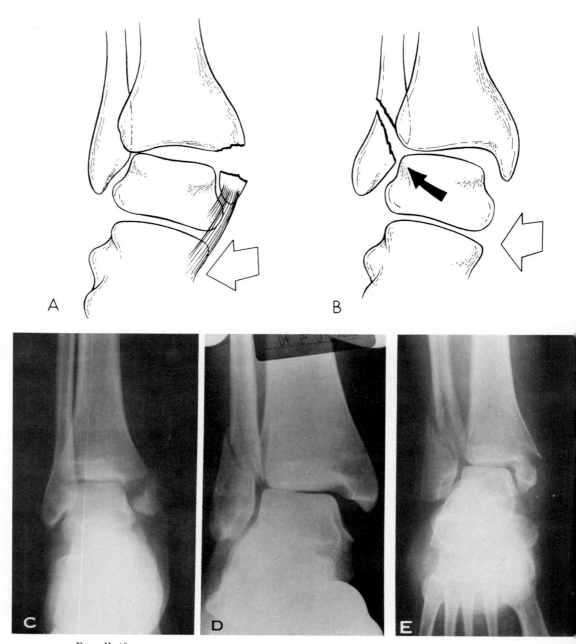

Fig. II.46.
  (A) Diagrammatic representation of an avulsion fracture of the medial malleolus.
  (B) Diagrammatic representation of an oblique fracture of the lateral malleolus produced by shearing force.
  (C) A transverse fracture of the medial malleolus caused by an avulsion force.
  (D) An oblique fracture of the lateral malleolus caused by a shearing force.
  (E) An avulsion fracture of the medial malleolus and shearing fracture of the lateral malleolus occurring simultaneously.

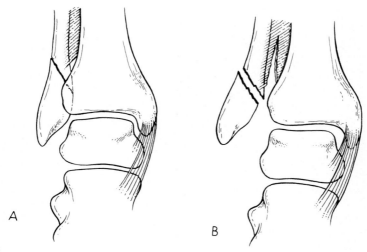

A   B

FIG. II.47.

(A) Fracture of the lateral malleolus occurring above its articular surface, thus the ankle mortise is not involved.

(B) Similar fracture as in (A), above the articular surface with disturbance of the mortise due to separation of the syndesmosis.

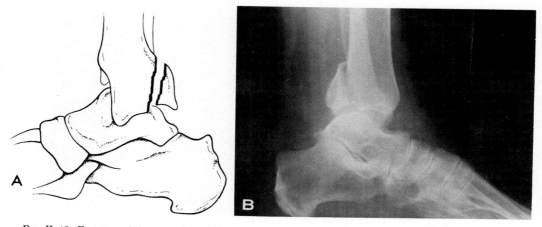

FIG. II.48. Fracture of the posterior malleolus.

(A) Diagrammatic representation.

(B) Radiograph. Note that approximately one-third of the articular surface is separated and displaced in a posterior and superior direction.

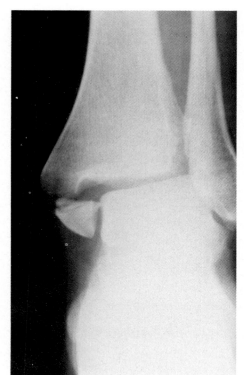

FIG. II.49. Bimalleolar fracture. The medial malleolus is being avulsed and the lateral malleolus is being fractured by a shearing force, resulting in a transverse fracture of the medial malleolus and an oblique fracture of the lateral malleolus.

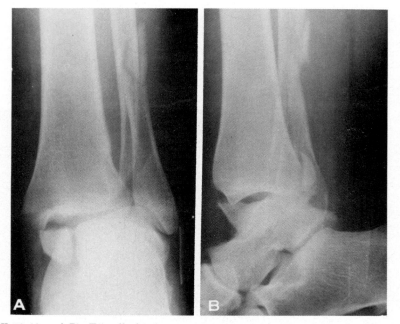

FIG. II.50 (A and B). Trimalleolar fracture. Anteroposterior (A) and lateral (B) radiographs demonstrate a transverse fracture of the medial malleolus and a long oblique comminuted fracture of the lateral malleolus. On the lateral projection, the small posterior malleolar fragment is seen in addition to the fractures of the medial and lateral malleoli.

duced is usually severely comminuted, producing various fracture patterns.

Anterior marginal fractures also occur, being produced by forceful dorsiflexion of the foot or anterior dislocation of the ankle, driving the talus against the tibia (see Fig. II.54, page 135).

These fractures of the distal tibia which involve the joint are described in the usual manner, in addition noting that they are intraarticular in nature (Fig. II.51).

Several common identifiable patterns occur with fractures of this area. These are T- or Y-shaped fractures. These fractures are described as intraarticular comminuted fractures, or T- or Y-shaped fractures of the distal tibia (Fig. II.52).

Separation of the Tibiofibular Syndesmosis

At times, usually in association with malleolar fractures, there is a rupture of the supporting ligaments of the distal tibiofibular syndesmosis. If this occurs, there is a separation of the syndesmosis and widening of the ankle mortise. Radiographically, the widened ankle mortise is readily visible on anteroposterior view, with loss of the overlapping shadow of the distal tibia and fibula. The outline of the fibular notch is also visible. This injury is described as a diastasis or separation of the distal tibiofibular syndesmosis, with a description of the associated fracture, if any is present (Fig. II.53).

Dislocations of the Ankle

A dislocation of the ankle is present when the dome of the talus is displaced from the ankle mortise. Although the dislocation of the ankle may occur without a fracture, this is not usually the rule. Most dislocations of the ankle are associated with fractures of the lateral, medial, or posterior malleolus, alone or in combination. Those that occur alone have accompanying ligamentous rupture.

A dislocation of the ankle is designated by the relation of the talus to the mortise of the ankle joint. The most common dislocation of the ankle is posterior. In this situation, the talus lies posterior to the ankle joint. Anterior dislocations, which are less common, are almost always accompanied by a fracture of the anterior margin of the articular surface of the tibia (Fig. II.54).

If a fracture accompanies a dislocation of the ankle, it is referred to as a fracture dislocation.

Fracture Dislocation of the Ankle

The ankle mortise is a closely knit unit combining the malleoli, the inferior tibial articular surface, and the talus held together by strong ligaments. Fractures which occur are usually accompanied by displace-

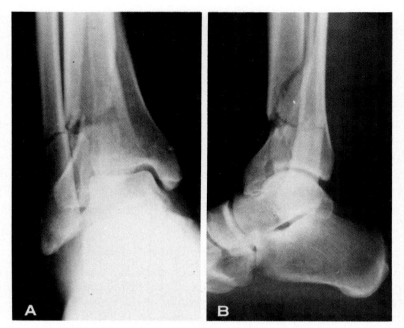

FIG. II.51 (A and B). Anteroposterior (A) and lateral (B) views of a comminuted intra-articular fracture of the distal tibia. Note the severe involvement of the ankle joint.

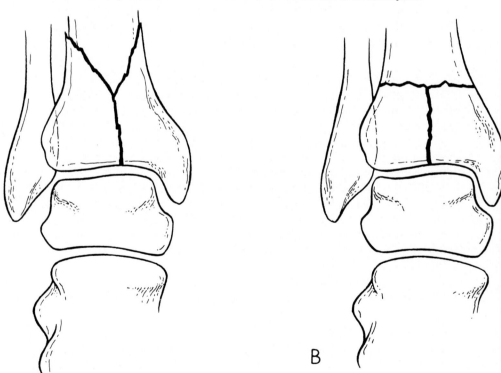

FIG. II.52.
    (A) Y-shaped comminuted intraarticular fracture of the distal tibia.
    (B) T-shaped comminuted intraarticular fracture of the distal tibia.

ment of the talus. These may range from minor displacement or subluxation to major or complete displacement or dislocation.

Fracture dislocations are probably more common than isolated dislocations without the presence of a fracture. These injuries are referred to as a fracture dislocation of the ankle and the description should include the components of the fracture as well as the direction of the dislocation (Fig. II.55).

Open or Compound Fractures or Fracture Dislocations of the Ankle

Since the bones of the ankle are so close to the skin, open injuries in this region are relatively frequent. Description of the ankle fracture is done in the conventional manner, by noting the nature of the injury, its location, direction, and other descriptive terms; for example, an open fracture or fracture dislocation of the ankle, naming the bones involved. Emphasis should be placed on the emergent nature of this injury in view of the possibility of sepsis.

Injuries to the Ankle in Children

Fractures about the ankle in children commonly involve the distal tibial epiphysis, and occur in any of the previously described forms for epiphyseal injuries. The injury can extend through the epiphyseal plate with displacement of the entire tibial epiphysis, with or without a metaphyseal fragment (Fig. II.56). Fractures also occur through the epiphyseal plate, at times, involving just the epiphysis of the medial malleolus (Fig. II.57). Falls from a height which produce intraarticular fractures in adults may produce crush injury to all or part of the epiphyseal plate in children, resulting in growth disturbance of the extremity.

These fractures are described in the usual manner for epiphyseal fractures.

Review

Identify the fractures illustrated (Figs. A-D). Correct identification is given on page 385.

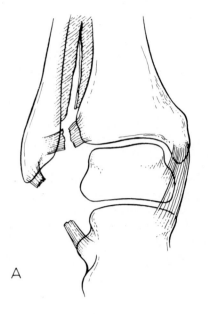

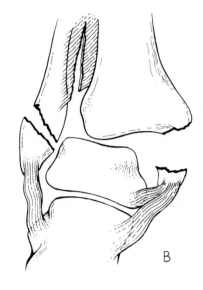

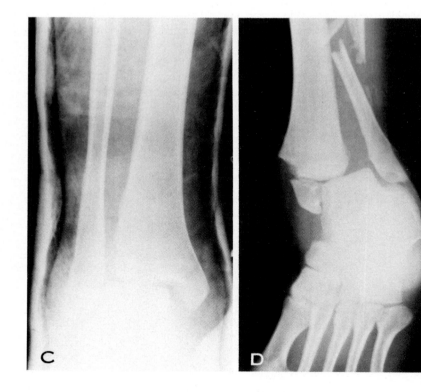

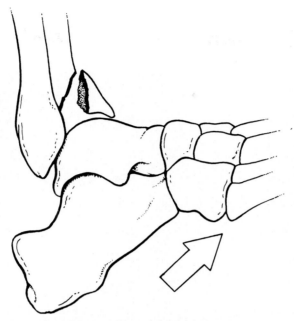

FIG. II.54. Anterior dislocation of the ankle, associated
with fracture of the anterior aspect of the tibia.

FIG. II.53. Separation of the distal tibiofibular syndesmosis.

   (A) Separation of the tibiofibular syndesmosis without an accompanying fracture.

   (B) Separation of the syndesmosis associated with fracture of the medial and lateral
malleoli.

   (C) Anteroposterior radiograph of a separation of the syndesmosis without an accompanying fracture. Note that the ankle mortise is widened and that there is no over-
laping shadow of the distal tibia and fibula.

   (D) A separation of the syndesmosis associated with fracture of the medial malleolus
and a comminuted fracture of the distal fibula.

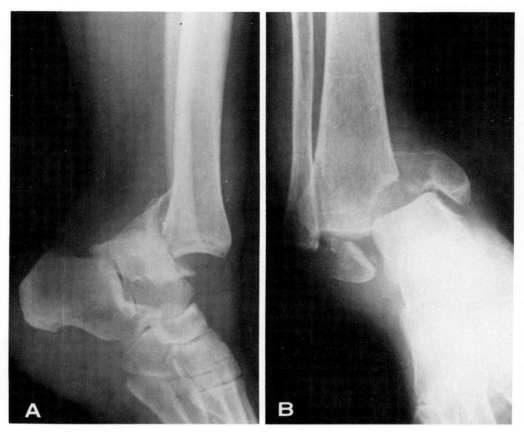

Fig. II.55.

(A) Posterior fracture dislocation of the ankle. Note the fracture of the medial malleolus, the lateral malleolus, and the posterior malleolus and that the talus has come to rest posterior to the ankle joint.

(B) Medial fracture dislocation of the ankle. In this case a fracture of the lateral malleolus and medial malleolus has occurred and the talus has come to rest medial to the ankle joint.

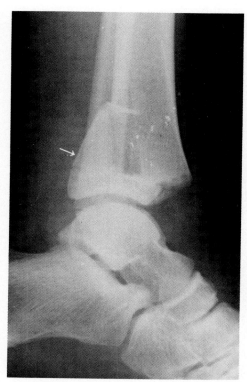

Fig. II.56. Fracture separation of the distal tibial epiphysis. Note that a segment of metaphysis has accompanied the epiphysis and there is posterior displacement of the epiphyseal fragment.

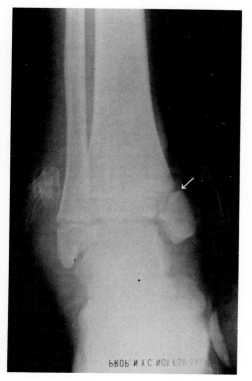

Fig. II.57. Fracture of the epiphysis of the medial malleolus.

Figs. A–D.

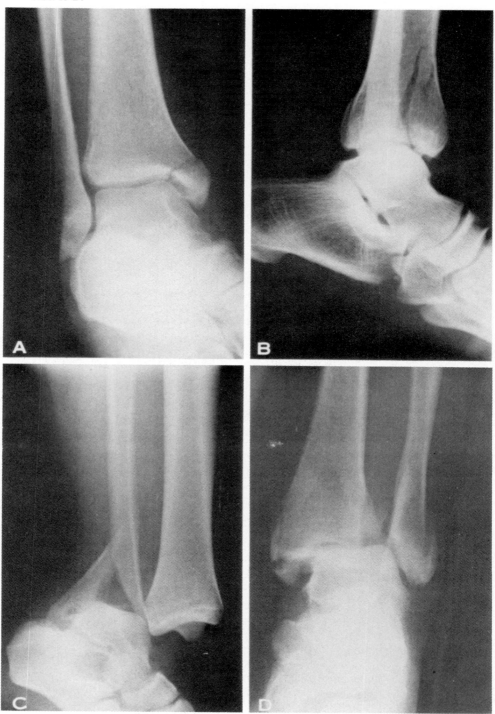

THE FOOT

ANATOMY

The foot is the contact point of the body in gait and structurally may be divided into three areas: a hindfoot, a midfoot, and a forefoot.

The hindfoot is composed of two large tarsal bones, the talus and the calcaneus (or os calcis), whereas the midfoot is composed of the remaining five tarsal bones, the navicular, cuboid, and the medial, intermediate, and lateral cuneiform bones. The forefoot is composed of the metatarsals and the phalanges of each of the five toes (Fig. II.58).

Ossification

Unlike the carpal bones whose ossification proceeds in a diagrammatic systematic spiral, the time of ossification of the tarsus, although relatively consistent in appearance, forms no easy pattern to remember.

Each tarsal bone is ossified from a single center except the calcaneus which has a separate epiphysis for its tuberosity. The calcaneus, talus, and cuboid of the tarsus are well ossified at the time of birth. The lateral cuneiform ossifies during the 1st year of life, the medial cuneiform during the 3rd year, and the intermediate cuneiform and navicular during the 4th year of life. The epiphysis of the tuberosity of the os calcis appears about the 5th to the 12th year (Fig. II.59).

Of the bones of the foot, the talus and the os calcis are the most interesting clinically and will be discussed separately.

THE TALUS

Anatomy

The talus (Fig. II.60) is a dome-shaped bone of irregular contour and, with the distal ends of the tibia and fibula, comprises the ankle joint. It is the only bone in the foot which does not provide attachments for any muscle but does serve for the attachment of several ligaments.

139

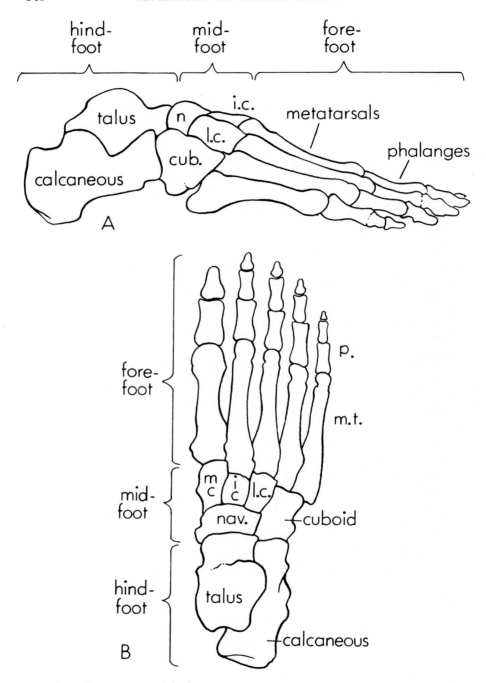

Fig. II.58. Bony anatomy of the foot.
  (A) Lateral side of foot.   (C) Lateral projection of radiograph of normal foot.
  (B) Foot from above.   (D) Anteroposterior projection of normal foot.

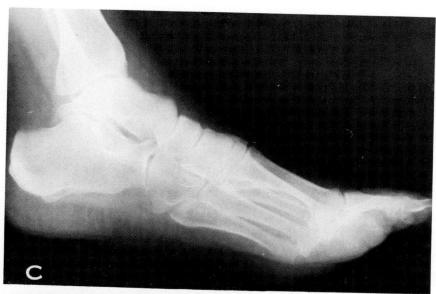

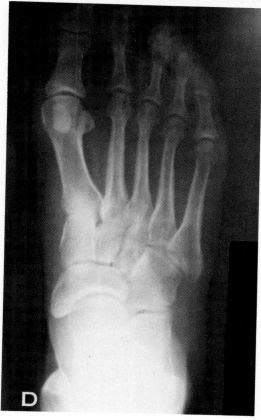

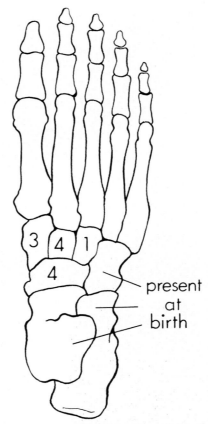

Fig. II.59. Age of ossification of tarsal bones in years.

For descriptive purposes, it is divided into a *head, neck,* and *body.* The head of the talus is the rounded anterior end of the bone which is covered by articular cartilage and joined to the body by a short, slightly constricted area called the neck. In the neck, there are foramina for the entrance of blood vessels. The body of the talus is irregular in shape and has several surfaces. The superior aspect, called the trochlea, is dome-shaped, covered by articular cartilage, and articulates with the tibia and fibula to form the ankle joint. It is wider in front than it is posteriorly and, therefore, fits snugly into the ankle mortise with dorsiflexion of the foot. The inferior surface of the body contains two concave articular facets to articulate with the os calcis. Between the two facets is a deep groove, the sulcus tali, which rests above a similar groove in the os calcis forming the sinus tarsi. Posteriorly, the talus is projected into a posterior process consisting of a medial and lateral tubercle which border a sulcus grooved for the tendon of the flexor hallucis longus.

The talus has several articulations. The superior prominence of the

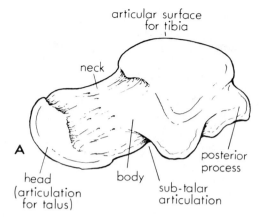

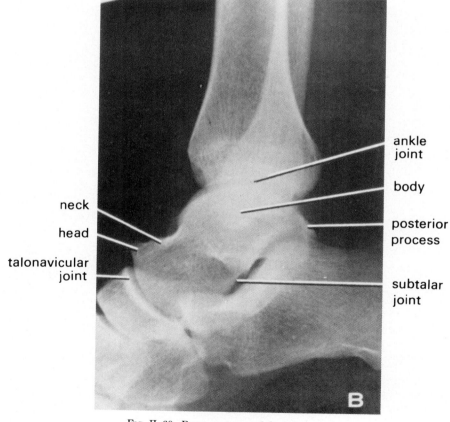

Fig. II.60. Bony anatomy of the talus.
(A) Diagram of the talus from the side.
(B) Lateral radiograph of the talus.

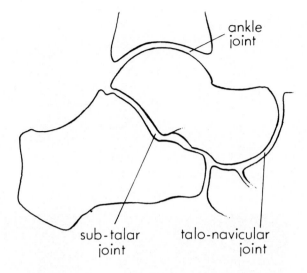

FIG. II.61. Talus and its articulations.

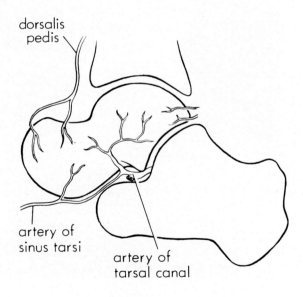

FIG. II.62. Blood supply of the talus.

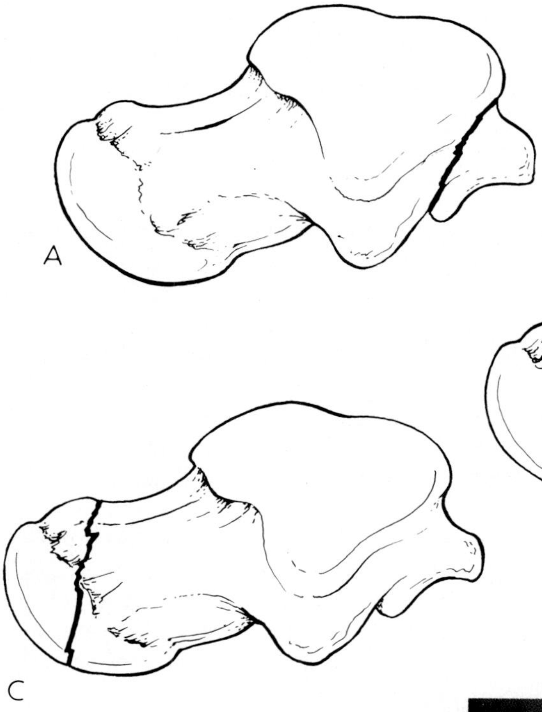

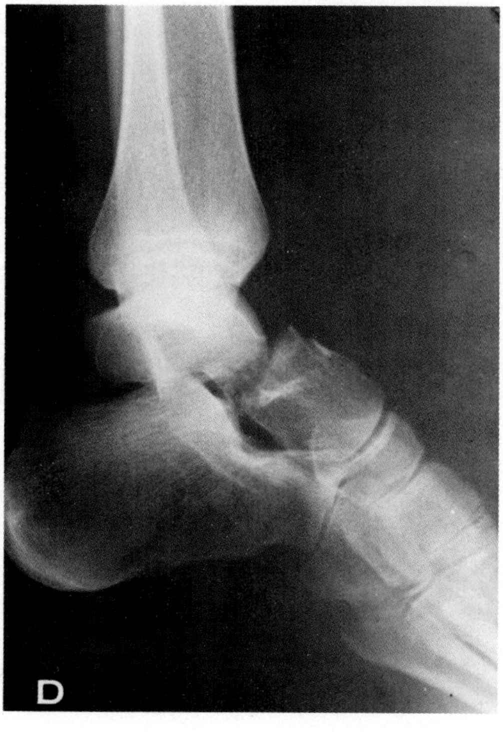

FIG. II.63. Fractures of the talus can be described by the anatomic area involved.

(A) Fracture of the posterior process.

(B) Fracture of the body.

(C) Fracture of the head.

(D) Radiograph of a transverse fracture of the body of the talus.

body, the dome, supports the tibia, forming the ankle joint, whereas the inferior aspect rests on the os calcis forming the subtalar joint. The anterior aspect of the talus articulates with the navicular forming the talonavicular joint (Figs. II.60 B and II.61).

Blood Supply (Fig. II. 62)

The arterial supply of the talus arises predominantly from branches of the anterior and posterior tibial arteries.

The posterior tibial artery distributes small branches to the posterior tubercle and then proceeds to make its major contribution via the artery of the tarsal canal, the largest branch of which enters the talus in the middle of the body.

Another branch of the artery of the tarsal canal passes between the deltoid ligament to supply the medial periosteal surface of the body and anastomosis with the dorsalis pedis artery over the neck of the talus.

The anterior tibial artery, becoming the dorsalis pedis artery, gives branches to the superior surface of the neck, but makes its major contribution by means of the artery of the sinus tarsi. The latter vessel also distributes branches to the head, but continues on to anastomose with the artery of the tarsal canal, which then enters the talus as described above.

The intraosseous pattern therefore is such that the head of the talus is supplied by the dorsalis pedis artery and branches of the artery of the sinus tarsi, whereas the body is supplied predominately by the artery of the tarsal canal following its anastomosis with the tarsal sinus artery.

NOMENCLATURE

Fractures

Fractures of the talus, although difficult to treat, are simple to describe, as our routine terms are applied to the anatomic area involved. Thus fractures may occur through the head, neck, body, or posterior process of the talus (Fig. II.63).

As most fractures of the talus extend into joints, they are, of course, intraarticular in nature and may be classified as such. Avulsion fractures also occur and are usually located anteriorly on the superior surface where the joint capsule inserts (Fig. II.64).

Dislocations

The talus, in addition to being predisposed to fractures, is, in view of its multiple articulations, also predisposed to dislocations. The dislocations may take place at any of the articular surfaces of the bone. Thus dislocations may take place at the ankle joint with the rest of the foot remaining in its proper anatomic position, at the subtalar joint (joint between the os calcis and talus), or anteriorly, at the talonavicular joint with the talus retaining its position in the mortise (Fig. II.65).

Any combination of dislocations may occur. A single area may be dislocated, as previously noted, or there may be two or more joints dislocated at the same time, for example, the body of the talus dislocated at the subtalar and the talonavicular joint. The most severe injury is total dislocation of the talus with disruption of all the articulations of the talus (Fig. II.66).

Consistent with our basic terminology, however, any combination of fractures or fracture dislocations may be readily described by first considering the joint or joints disturbed, be it the ankle joint, subtalar joint, or talonavicular joint and, secondly, the nature, location, and direction of any accompanying fractures, if present (Fig. II.67).

Complications of Fractures and Dislocations of the Talus

The complications of fractures and dislocations of the talus are mainly concerned with avascular necrosis of the body of the talus.

Avascular Necrosis

The talus is one of several bones which include the femoral head, the carpal navicular and the lunate, which because of the nature of their

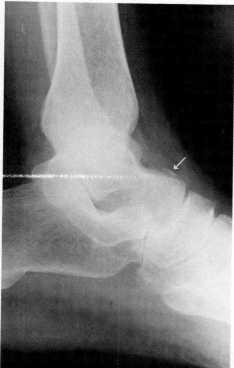

Fig. II.64. Avulsion fracture of the anterior superior surface of the talus.

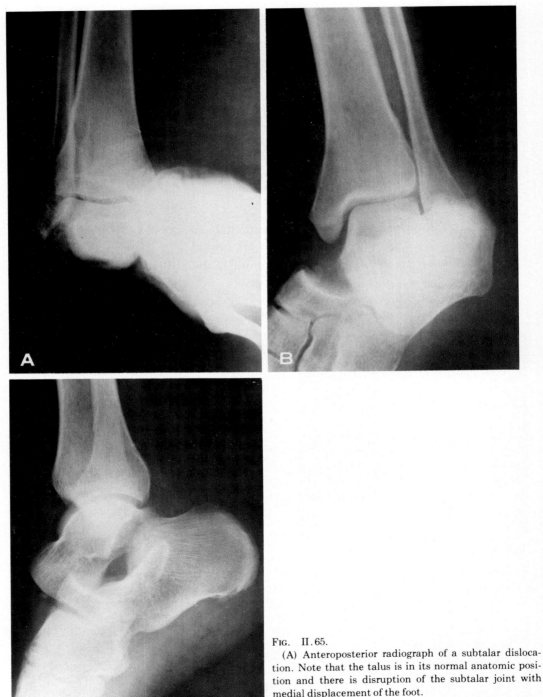

Fig.   II.65.

(A) Anteroposterior radiograph of a subtalar dislocation. Note that the talus is in its normal anatomic position and there is disruption of the subtalar joint with
medial displacement of the foot.

(B) Anteroposterior view of a combined talonavicular
and subtalar dislocation.

(C) Lateral view of dislocation shown in (B).

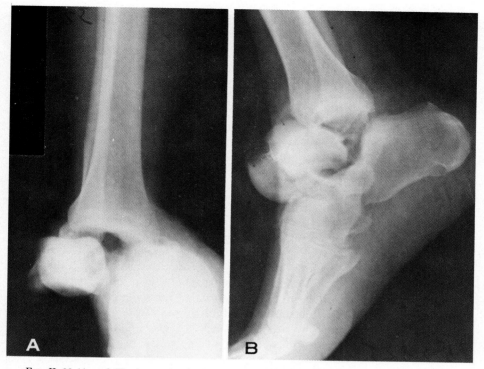

FIG. II.66 (A and B). Anteroposterior (A) and lateral (B) radiographs of a total dislocation of the talus.

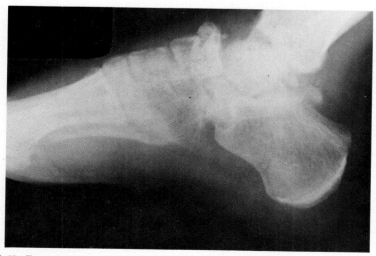

FIG. II.67. Fracture dislocation. Fracture through the body of the talus with dislocation of the head of the talus.

blood supply, is predisposed to avascular necrosis following trauma (see "Blood Supply," page 146). Avascular necrosis occurs in the body of the talus when fractures occur through the neck or dislocations occur which involve the subtalar joint, causing interruption of the blood supply to the body of the talus. The complication arises depending on the location of the fracture in relation to the entrance of the artery of the tarsal canal into the talus. Fractures occurring distal to the entrance of the artery do not interrupt the circulation to the bone, and thus both fragments remain well vascularized. Fractures occurring posterior to the entrance of the artery of the tarsal canal, however, interrupt the major blood supply to the body and predispose it to avascular necrosis. Dislocations which involve the subtalar joint can cause rupture of the artery of the tarsal canal and result in compromise of the circulation to the talus (Fig. II.68).

As with avascular necrosis, in general, radiologically, the bony architecture initially remains unchanged and the involved area becomes relatively more dense following a period of many months. Eventually there may be flattening of the dome of the talus, resulting in joint incongruities. Thus x-rays should be taken at intervals over an extended period of time in order to demonstrate the pathology manifested by increased density of the body of the talus (Fig. II.69). Fracture healing can take place despite the presence of avascular necrosis.

OS CALCIS (CALCANEUS)
Anatomy

The os calcis or heel bone, a major weight-bearing structure, is the largest bone of the foot and, with the talus, forms the hindfoot (Fig. II.70).

Arbitrarily, the os calcis may be divided into thirds: an anterior, middle, and posterior third as we have done previously with other bones. The anterosuperior two-thirds support the talus, and with it form the subtalar joint, whereas the posteroinferior third forms the prominence of the heel and rests on the ground.

The anterior aspect of the superior surface of the os calcis contains three facets for articulation with the talus. A deep depression is present between the facets called the calcaneal sulcus which is located beneath the sulcus tali, forming the sinus tarsi. The posterior aspect of the superior surface is nonarticular and extends to the tuberosity.

On the posteroinferior surface is the tuberosity which is the posterior prominence of the calcaneus, and a major weight-bearing area. It is nonarticular and serves for the insertion of the Achilles tendon. Medially a horizontally projecting shelf is located at about the level of the junction of the anterior and middle third of the os calcis, the sustentaculum tali, which contains an articular facet and acts to support the talus (Fig. II.71).

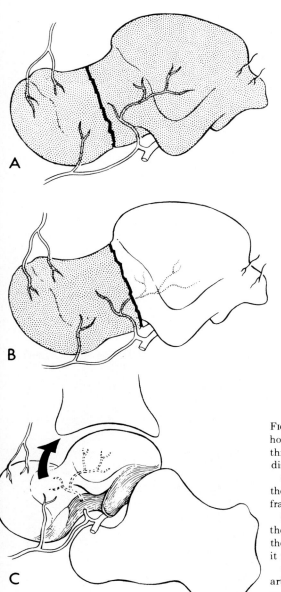

Fig. II.68. Blood supply to the talus demonstrating how disruption of the subtalar joint and fractures through the neck can interrupt the arterial supply, predisposing the bone to avascular necrosis.

(A) Fractures occurring anterior to the entrance of the artery of the tarsal canal into the talus permit both fragments to be well vascularized.

(B) Fractures occurring posterior to the entrance of the artery of the tarsal canal into the talus interrupts the major blood supply to the body, thus predisposing it to avascular necrosis.

(C) Subtalar dislocations can cause rupture of the artery of the tarsal canal and, in this way, interrupt the vascularity of the body of the talus, leading to avascular necrosis.

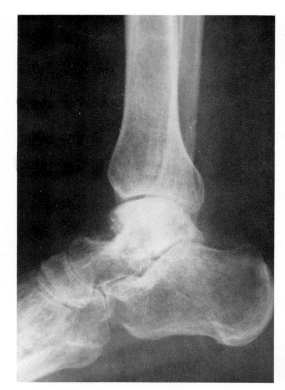

Fig. II.69 Avascular necrosis of the talus following fracture through the body. The body of the talus is relatively more dense than the surrounding bone. Note that the fracture has healed.

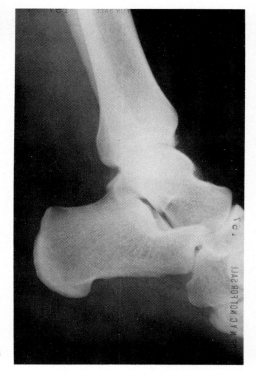

Fig. II.70. Lateral radiograph of a normal os calcis and its articulations.

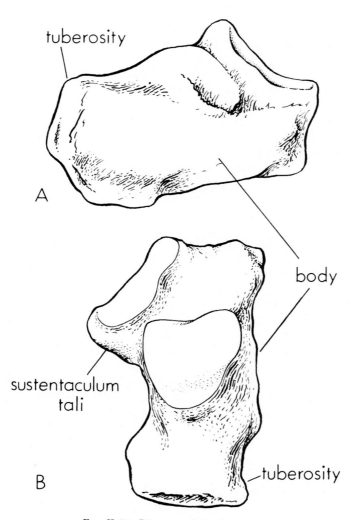

FIG. II.71. Diagram of the bony anatomy of the os calcis.
    (A) Lateral side of os calcis.
    (B) Os calcis from above.

Fractures of the Os Calcis

Fractures of the calcaneus occur as a result of direct severe impact, as with a fall from a height, or may be of an avulsion type, occurring secondary to the strong pull of the Achilles tendon.

The site of fractures of the os calcis may be described simply by the arbitrary reference points established, as being located in the anterior, middle, or posterior thirds, and the direction by the pattern of the fracture line in conjunction with our basic principles. There are, however, two basic major considerations which must be made in describing fractures of the os calcis. These are:

1. Fractures which do not enter the subtalar joint.
2. Fractures which extend into the subtalar joint.

As the expected prognosis in these are significantly different, with the intraarticular fractures having a much more serious outlook, distinction is of more than academic interest.

Thus, in general, fractures of the os calcis are described by the location of the fracture, the direction and amount of comminution of the fracture, and the presence or absence of subtalar joint involvement.

Fractures Which Do Not Enter the Subtalar Joint

Extraarticular fractures are those fractures which involve the posterior third of the os calcis or the tuberosity. These fractures are usually produced by a fall from a height onto the heels and result in a bursting type of injury, with severe comminution and many directions of fracture lines. Also, extraarticular fractures are produced by severe violent contracture of the triceps surae muscles or violent dorsiflexion injury to the foot, resulting in an avulsion fracture of the tuberosity which serves as the attachment of the Achilles tendon.

Despite the severe appearance of some of these fractures, extraarticular fractures may be described in our routine fashion as to the location of the fracture, the direction of the fracture, the presence of comminution, or the presence of avulsed fragments (Fig. II.72).

Intraarticular Fractures

Intraarticular fractures are those in which the fracture line extends into and involves the subtalar joint. These fractures may range from a single fracture line to ones with marked comminution.

The shape of the superior surface of the os calcis, viewed on lateral projection, allows for the formation of a relatively fixed angle. This angle is formed by the projection of a straight line from the tuberosity to the dome, with a second line from the dome along the subtalar joint to the tip of the anterior aspect of the os calcis. This angle is known as Boehler's tuber-joint angle and is normally approximately 20–40°.

With crush injuries or displaced intraarticular involvement of the

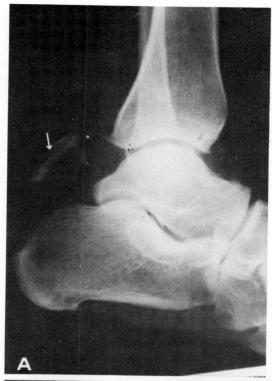

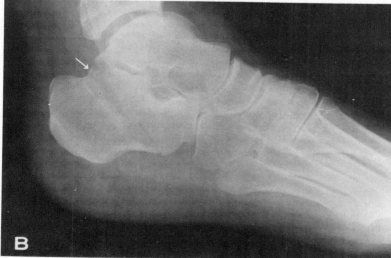

Fig. II.72.

(A) Avulsion fracture of the tuberosity. Note the distraction caused by the pull of the gastrocnemius-soleus group of muscles, and that the subtalar joint is not involved.

(B) Oblique fracture through the middle third of the os calcis. Note that the fracture does not enter the subtalar joint.

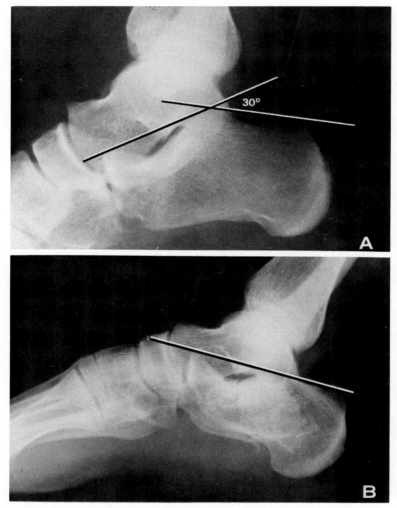

FIG. II.73. Boehler's tuber-joint angle.
  (A) Intersecting lines forming Boehler's angle are normally approximately 20–40°.
  (B) Comminuted intraarticular fracture. Note the decrease in Boehler's angle.

subtalar joint, this angle is decreased, being reduced at times to even a negative angle. Measurement of this angle may assist in diagnosis of fractures of the os calcis (Fig. II.73). Extraarticular fractures can also have alteration in the tuber-joint if the posterior aspect is displaced upward.

Although fractures involving the subtalar joint can appear quite comminuted and the x-ray appearance quite complicated, the description is relatively simple with application of our basic principles, and may simply be classified as an intraarticular fracture of the anterior third, body, or middle third of the os calcis. The direction, comminution, displacement, and nature of the fracture may be described as indicated (Fig. II.74).

Another type of intraarticular fracture occurs at the anterosuperior aspect of the os calcis and is usually the result of an avulsion force. These fractures are simply designated by the site of the pathology, as an intraarticular fracture of the anterosuperior margin of the os calcis (Fig. II.75).

THE MIDFOOT

Fractures

The rest of the tarsal bones are relatively square or rectangular in shape, and fractures occurring through these bones occur either as avulsion fractures or by direct trauma resulting in comminuted fractures. These injuries may be described in routine fashion, noting the bone involved and applying the other descriptive terms as indicated (Fig. II.76).

Dislocations

In addition to dislocation about the talus, dislocation may involve the os calcis as well as the intertarsal joints. These injuries are simply described by the bones and joints involved (Fig. II.77).

THE FOREFOOT

Fractures

Fractures of the metatarsals and phalanges are described in the usual manner for long bones, with arbitrary division into thirds (proximal, middle, or distal thirds) and by the direction, angulation, as well as whether they are open or closed. At times, however, fractures of the metatarsals and phalanges may be described by anatomic location. Thus, fractures that are just proximal to the head of the metatarsals or phalanges may be described as fractures through the neck; fractures in the proximal third of the metatarsals and phalanges may be described as fractures at the base (Fig. II.78).

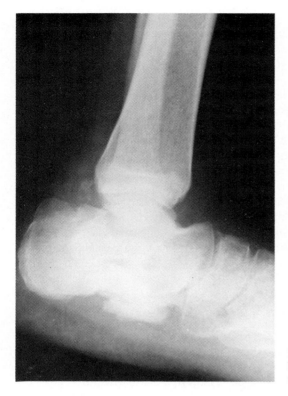

Fig. II.74. Comminuted intraarticular fracture of the body of the os calcis. Note the marked flattening of the anterior aspect of the os calcis.

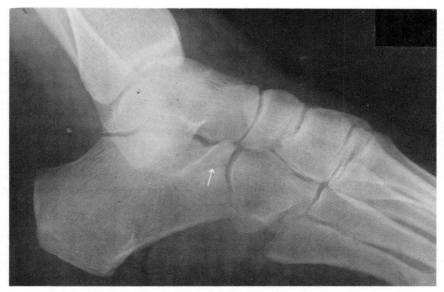

Fig. II.75. Intraarticular fracture of the anterosuperior aspect of the os calcis.

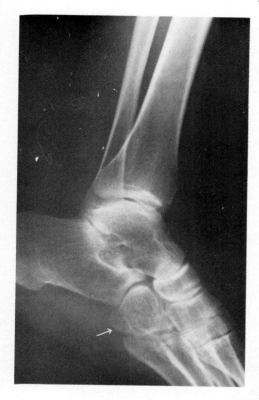

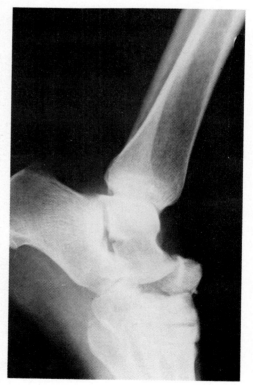

FIG. II.76. Comminuted fracture of the cuboid.

FIG. II.77. Dorsal dislocation of the navicular. Note
that there is also a fracture through the body of the talus.

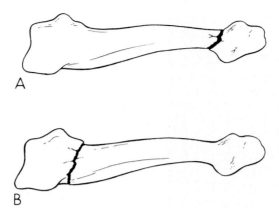

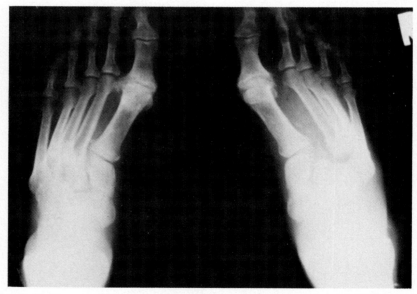

Fig. II.78.
(A) Fracture of the head of a metatarsal.
(B) Fracture of the base of a metatarsal.

Fig. II.79. Fracture dislocation of the tarsal-metatarsal joint of the second through the fifth metatarsals with lateral displacement of the metatarsals on the right. The opposite extremity is shown for comparison.

Dislocations

Tarsometatarsal joint, metatarsal phalangeal joint, and interphalangeal joint dislocations may occur and are described by the joint and digit involved and the final position of the distal bone in relation to the proximal one (Fig. II.79). For example, if the middle phalanx of the third toe is dislocated dorsally, it would be described as a dorsal dislocation of the proximal interphalangeal joint of the third toe. Dislocations are usually dorsal or volar at the interphalangeal and metatarsal phalangeal joints and lateral at the tarsal metatarsal joints.

AVULSION FRACTURES

Avulsion fractures may involve any of the bones of the tarsus, metatarsus, and phalanges, and these are described in routine fashion as avulsion fractures of the involved bone and area.

FATIGUE FRACTURES

(See "Stress Fracture," page 30.)

Metatarsals

Of all the bones in the body, the metatarsals are the most frequently involved with fatigue fractures or stress fractures. A common eponym used is a *march fracture* (see "March Fracture," page 314). March fractures refer basically to lesions of the metatarsals and are a result of repeated submaximal stresses to an otherwise normal bone which eventually result in local bony change and finally fracture. The injury is found most commonly in military personnel and the second metatarsal is the bone most frequently involved, followed closely by the third metatarsal. The first and fifth metatarsals are rarely affected. Initial x-ray examinations at the onset of symptoms are usually normal; however, they become diagnostic 2–14 days later. These fractures are described by the usual methods as to location, direction, and bone involved.

Os Calcis

Fatigue fractures of the os calcis, although not common, do occur due to repetitive impact upon the bone. The type of fatigue fracture seen in the os calcis is that of the compression variety. X-ray confirmation of this injury takes longer than that for metatarsals, averaging about 5 weeks after the onset of symptoms. The initial x-ray finding is sclerosis. Displacement of fracture fragments almost never occurs (Fig. II.80).

Review

Identify the fractures illustrated (Figs. A–F). Correct identification is given on page 386.

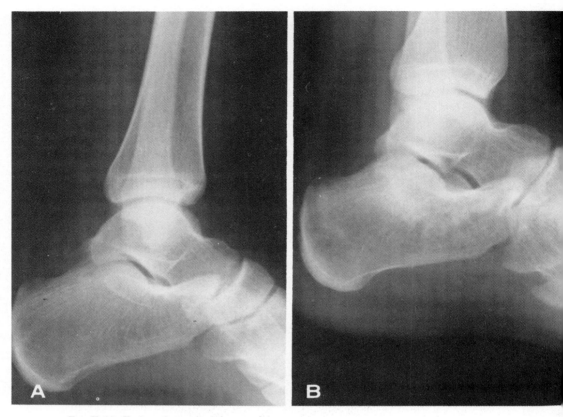

FIG. II.80. Fatigue fracture of the os calcis.
    (A) X ray of os calcis at onset of symptoms.
    (B) Six weeks later. Note the increased density (sclerosis) below the anterosuperior surface.

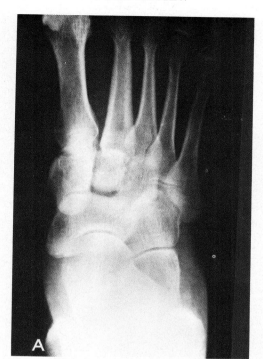

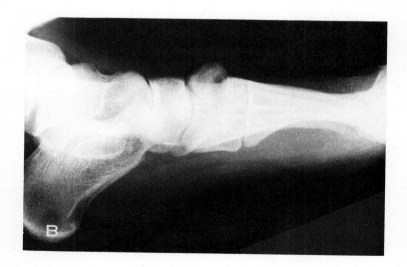

164

Figs. C–F.

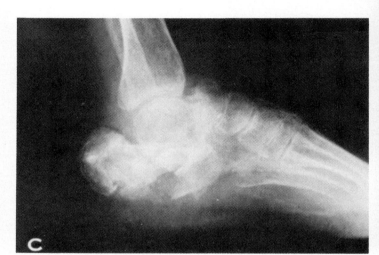

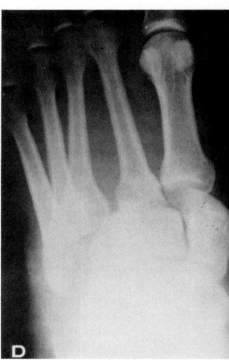

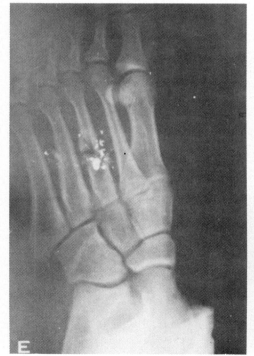

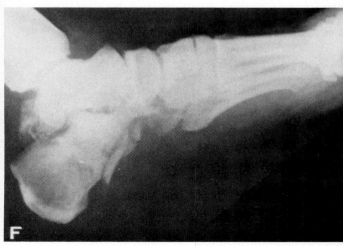

SPINE

ANATOMY

The vertebral column is composed of 33 vertebrae arranged in longitudinal fashion and articulated with one another. Articulation between vertebrae occurs in two locations, posteriorly by the small articular facets and anteriorly by fibrocartilaginous intervertebral discs (Fig. II.81). The vertebral column is divided into areas, the cervical with 7 vertebrae, the thoracic with 12, the lumbar region with 5, the 5 sacral, and 4 coccygeal vertebrae.

Other than at the two extremes of the vertebral column, namely the first and second cervical vertebrae and the sacrum and coccygeal vertebrae, the other vertebrae, although slightly different in size and shape, have basic general characteristics which make them similar to each other (Fig. II.82). The vertebrae may be anatomically divided into two sections, an *anterior element* called the body of the vertebrae and a *posterior element* formed by the vertebral arch which surrounds the spinal canal.

The body or anterior component of the vertebrae is large, thickened, and somewhat oval in shape, with a cartilaginous plate on its superior and inferior surfaces. The upper and lower surfaces are flattened. The bodies are articulated by a series of symphyses, being separated from one another by a fibrocartilaginous intervertebral disc.

The vertebral arch is composed of two pedicles which project backward from the dorsal aspect of the body and two laminae which project posteromedially from the pedicles, and meet in the midline. The pedicles are short and thick and have constrictions on the top and bottom, forming a shallow superior and a deep inferior vertebral notch. These notches, when combined in the articulated vertebrae, form the intervertebral foramina through which the spinal nerves run. The pedicles and laminae combine with the body to form a ring, enclosing the spinal canal through which the spinal cord runs. Attached to the vertebral arch are several projections, some of which serve for the attachment of muscles and ligaments, and others for articulation with other vertebrae.

165

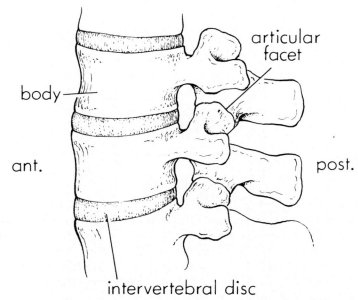

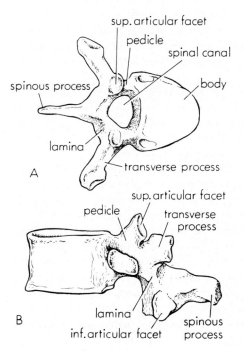

FIG. II.81. Articulations between vertebrae occur anteriorly by intervertebral fibrocartilaginous discs located between the bodies and posteriorly by articular facets connecting the posterior elements.

FIG. II.82. General characteristic bony anatomy of a vertebra:
(A) Vertebra from above.
(B) Vertebra from the side.

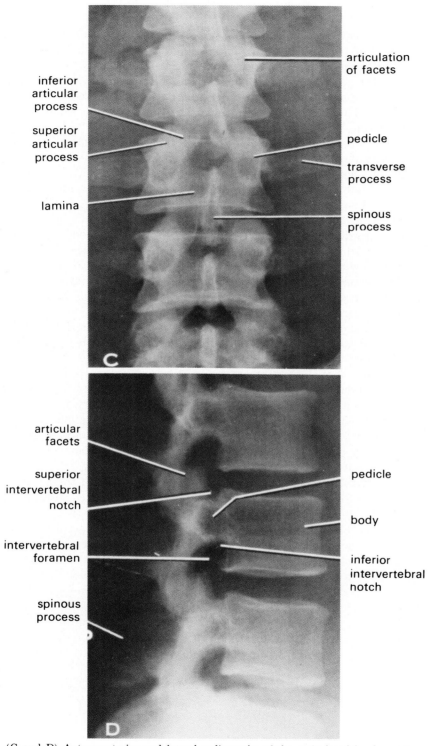

inferior
articular
process

superior
articular
process

lamina

articulation
of facets

pedicle

transverse
process

spinous
process

articular
facets

superior
intervertebral
notch

intervertebral
foramen

spinous
process

pedicle

body

inferior
intervertebral
notch

(C and D) Anteroposterior and lateral radiographs of the articulated lumbar spine.

The transverse processes are projections which are located at the junction of the pedicles and laminae, project laterally, and serve primarily for the attachments of muscles and ligaments. Also at the junction of the pedicles and laminae are two superior and two inferior articular processes, the apposing surfaces of which are covered with hyaline cartilage. The spinous process projects posteriorly from the junction of the laminae.

Variations in the characteristics of vertebrae from the basic anatomical pattern occur in certain locations. The *first cervical* vertebra (atlas) (Fig. II.83, lower) is essentially an oval ring without a body or a spinous process, and consists of an anterior and posterior arch and two lateral masses. The skull is supported by the lateral masses, and thus the term, the atlas.

The anterior arch forms approximately one-fifth of the ring. The posterior aspect of the anterior arch is concave and has a facet for the articulation with the odontoid process of the second cervical vertebra.

The posterior arch encloses the large spinal foramen and has, as its most dorsal projection, a rudiment of the spinous process, the posterior tubercle.

The *second cervical* vertebra (Fig. II.83, upper) or axis is also formed by an anterior and posterior segment. Its main variation is located anteriorly where there is a perpendicular, superiorly directed projection of bone called the odontoid process. On the anterior aspect of the odontoid is a facet, against which the facet of the posterior aspect of the anterior arch of the atlas articulates, allowing for rotary movement of the head. The dorsal surface of the odontoid has a shallow groove to accommodate the transverse atlantal ligament. The posterior segment of the axis, like the other vertebrae, is composed of the pedicles and laminae, in addition to transverse and spinous processes.

The articulation of the atlas with the axis consists of three joints, a pivot joint between the odontoid and the anterior arch, and gliding joints at the two lateral atlantal axial articulations. At the junction of the anterior arch and the odontoid are two synovial cavities, one between the posterior surface of the anterior arch and the odontoid, and the other between the transverse atlantal ligament and the odontoid. Several ligaments contribute to the stability of the articulation, the most important of which is the transverse atlantal ligament. This ligament is a thick band attached to the medial surfaces of the lateral masses, and spans across the odontoid, keeping it in contact with the anterior arch of the atlas. Rupture of this ligament can produce dislocation of the vertebrae and spinal cord compression (see Fig. II.96, p. 183).

The sacrum is also a variant, consisting of the fusion of five vertebrae

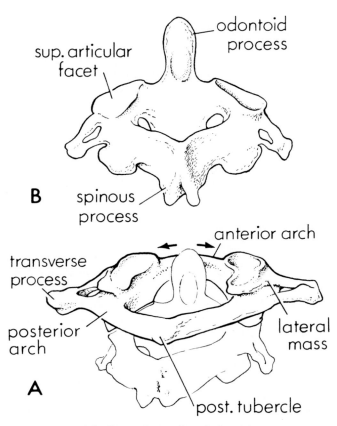

FIG. II.83. Bony anatomy of the first and second cervical vertebrae.
(A) First cervical vertebra and its relationship to C-2. Note that the vertebra is essentially a ring. Rotary motion of the head occurs by rotation of the axis about the odontoid.
(B) Axis (C-2) is unique only by the presence of the odontoid.

into a broadened triangular shaped irregular bone with a pelvic and dorsal surface. It is situated at the lower part of the vertebral column, articulating with the fifth lumbar vertebra and set inbetween the two innominate bones. Its inferior margin articulates with the coccyx. The coccyx is composed of a row of four small, slightly circular shaped rudimentary vertebrae.

The articulated longitudinal arrangement of the vertebral column is supported by various ligaments and forms four basic curves, namely a cervical lordotic curve, a thoracic kyphotic curve, a lumbar lordotic curve, and a sacral kyphosis (Fig. II.84). This is to say that the cervical vertebrae form an anterior curve with its concavity posteriorly, whereas the thoracic vertebrae form a posterior curve with its concavity anteriorly. The lumbar curve, like the cervical curve, is an anterior curve with its concavity posteriorly, and the sacrum and the coccyx, like the thoracic curve, have their concavity anteriorly.

The articulation of the vertebral column consists of a series of symphyses between the vertebral bodies and synovial joints between the vertebral arches. The joints of the vertebral arches are of the gliding variety, enclosed in an articular capsule and lined with a synovial membrane. The capsule is loose, being attached to the margins of the articular processes of adjacent vertebrae, and does not provide stability.

The stability of the vertebral column is provided by various ligaments. Extending the full length of the vertebral column are the strong anterior, longitudinal, and posterior longitudinal ligaments, in contact with the anterior and posterior surfaces of the bodies of the vertebrae. Additional stability is produced by ligaments attached to the vertebral arches and its projections, namely the ligamentum flavum, supraspinal ligaments, ligamentum nuchae, interspinal ligaments, and intertransverse ligaments.

INJURIES OF THE VERTEBRAL COLUMN

Fractures and dislocations of the spine may occur in various forms according to the nature of the trauma. For example, sections of the vertebrae may be compressed while other areas may be involved in linear or avulsion fractures.

Therefore, based on the anatomy, we may establish five component areas to apply our fracture vocabulary:

1. The body.
2. The pedicles.
3. The laminae.
4. The spinous and tranverse processes.
5. The intervertebral area.

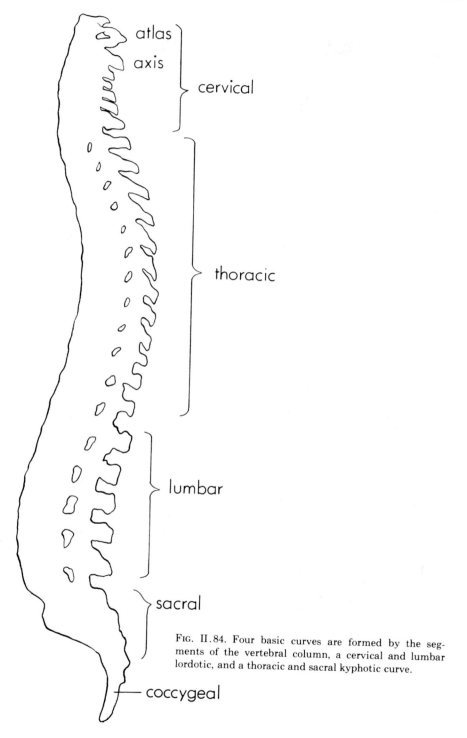

atlas
axis
cervical
thoracic
lumbar
sacral
coccygeal

FIG. II.84. Four basic curves are formed by the segments of the vertebral column, a cervical and lumbar lordotic, and a thoracic and sacral kyphotic curve.

FRACTURES OF THE SPINE

Although classification of injuries of the spine may appear quite complicated because of the multiple bones which compose the vertebral column, descriptions of fractures of the spine are simply applications of our usual terminology to the various anatomic areas.

Thus fractures of the spine may be divided into fractures of the bodies, fractures of the laminae, fractures of the pedicles, and fractures of the transverse and spinous processes. Furthermore, the description of these fractures must take into account the level of the injury, designating the vertebrae involved. Further elaboration should take into account the direction of the fracture.

It should be mentioned that fracture of the bony elements of the spine in itself is not a dangerous injury. It may, however, become a significant pathologic entity because of its close association with the spinal cord and the potential for injury to the spinal cord and nerve roots.

Fractures of the Body (Anterior Element)

Fractures of the body of the vertebrae are those fractures which involve the anterior aspect of the vertebrae or the body of the vertebrae. These fractures are either wedge-shaped compression fractures, partial compression fractures, vertical fractures, avulsion fractures, or bursting or comminuted fractures.

The majority of fractures of the body of vertebrae are those of the compression type which are caused when the spine is hyperflexed (Fig. II.85). In this injury, an impaction or compression of the anterior aspect of the vertebrae occurs, and the body of the vertebrae can assume a wedge-shaped appearance with the narrow aspect anteriorly, or have only a segment of the surface fractured, in which case the basic architecture of the vertebrae is unaltered. These fractures are simply described as a compression fracture of the body, noting the area of the body involved, displacement if present, and designating which vertebra is involved (Fig. II.86).

Linear vertical fractures also occur, more commonly in the cervical spine, but at times in the lumbar region. These fractures are described as vertical fractures of the body of the involved vertebrae.

The vertebral body is also subject to avulsion fractures, which occur when a segment of the body of the vertebra is avulsed by the supporting ligaments. These fractures are simply described by routine terminology, noting that they are avulsion fractures, further designating the surface of the body involved, as anterior, posterior, or lateral, and if it is superior or inferior, and designating the particular vertebra involved (Fig. II.87).

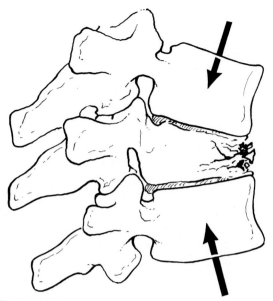

FIG. II.85. Compression fracture of the body of a vertebra occurs by flexion forces applied to the spine.

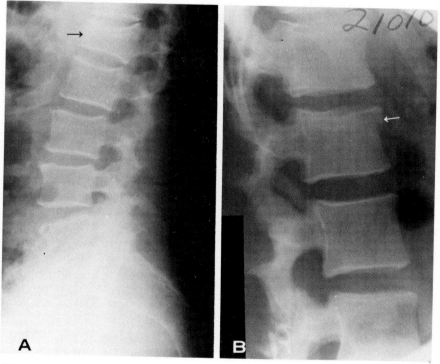

FIG. II.86. Compression fractures.
(A) Wedge-shaped compression fracture of the body of L-1.
(B) Compression fracture involving only the anterosuperior margin of the body of the vertebra.

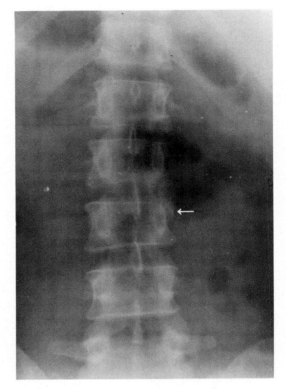

FIG. II.87. Avulsion fracture of the superolateral margin of the body of L-3.

Fracture of the Vertebral Arch (Posterior Elements)

Pedicles and Laminae

Fractures of the pedicles and laminae are usually produced by direct trauma and have particular significance inasmuch as the stability of the spine may be jeopardized. One or both pedicles or laminae may be fractured. These fractures are simply described, however, by the location and the direction of the fracture, and designating the vertebrae involved, such as transverse fracture of the pedicle of L-1 (Fig. II.88).

Articular Facets

Fractures of the articular facets are relatively rare lesions and are best seen on oblique x-ray projections. The injury may be unilateral or bilateral, and is described by the facet and vertebrae involved. Fracture of the articular facets adversely affects the stability of the spine and presents the potential for traumatic involvement of the spinal cord or nerve roots.

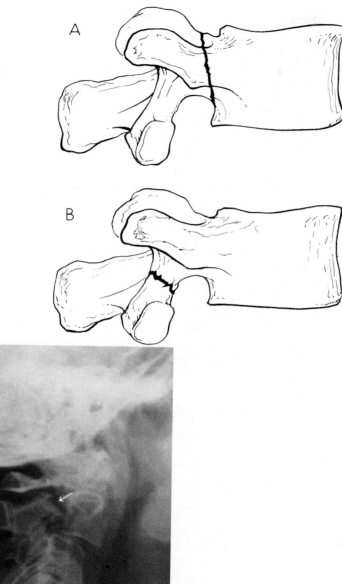

FIG. II.88. Diagrammatic representations of spinal fractures.

(A) Fracture through the pedicle.

(B) Fracture through the lamina.

(C) Radiograph of a transverse fracture of the pedicle of C-2. (Note the forward displacement of the body of C-2, indicating loss of stability due to the fracture.)

Transverse Processes

Fractures of the transverse processes are usually caused by severe muscular contraction, avulsing the transverse processes from their normal anatomic position. These fractures most commonly occur in the lumbar region and are described as avulsion fractures of the transverse process of the particular vertebra involved (Fig. II.89).

Spinous Process

Fractures of the spinous process usually occur by two mechanisms, direct violence, resulting in a comminuted fracture, or muscular violence, resulting in an avulsion force dislodging a fragment of bone. Again the terminology is simple, applying our routine vocabulary to the particular vertebrae involved.

VARIATIONS IN NOMENCLATURE

There are certain fractures of the spine which, because of their specific anatomic location, have specific terminology.

Fractures of the Atlas (C-1)

Fractures of the atlas are usually caused by a compression type injury, resulting in fracture of a segment or comminution of the ring of the atlas. These fractures are named for the area of the arch involved, be it anterior or posterior, the direction of the fracture line, and comminution noted, if present (Fig. II.90) (see "Jefferson Fracture," page 308).

Fractures of the Odontoid Process (DENS)

A fracture which involves the anterosuperior projection of the second cervical vertebra is designated by its anatomic location and is described as an odontoid fracture. As the odontoid process and the transverse atlantal ligament are the major stabilizing elements of the articulation of the atlas and axis, fracture of the odontoid is frequently accompanied by dislocation of C-1 on C-2. These fractures are difficult to visualize on routine anteroposterior radiographs and may be best seen on open mouth anteroposterior views (Fig. II.91). Lateral radiographs must also be taken to evaluate the fracture. Fractures of the odontoid process of C-2 are described by the direction of the fracture, the area of the odontoid involved, be it the base, midportion, or superior aspect, and the presence or absence of displacement should be noted (Fig. II.92). These fractures are extremely dangerous because of their close proximity to the spinal cord, their inherent instability, and the high level of the spinal cord lesion, which could result in the death of the patient.

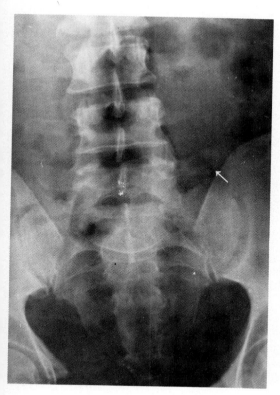

Fig. II.89. Avulsion fracture of the transverse process of L-5.

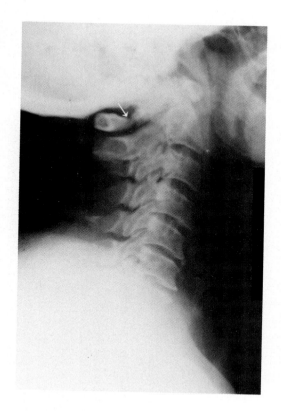

Fig. II.90. Transverse fracture of the posterior arch of C-1.

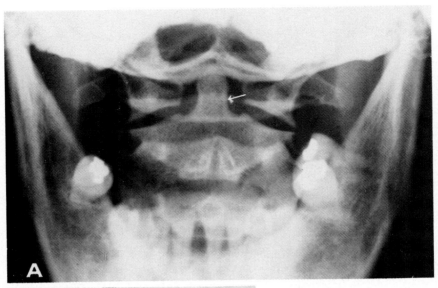

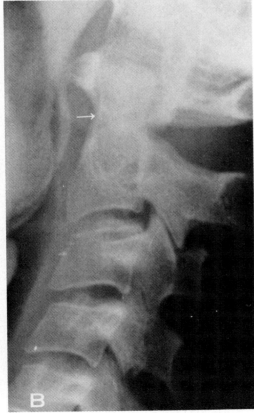

Fig. II.91. Normal odontoid.

(A) The Odontoid is best demonstrated in the anteroposterior plane through an open mouth view.

(B) Lateral view of odontoid.

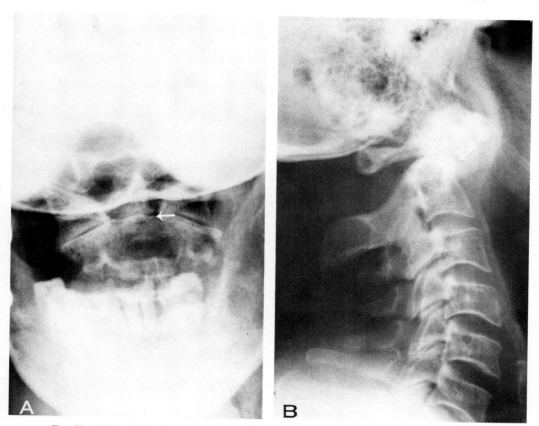

FIG. II.92 (A and B). Fracture of the odontoid with forward subluxation of C-1 on C-2. Anteroposterior open mouth (A) and lateral (B) views of a transverse fracture of the odontoid. Note on the lateral view the forward subluxation of C-1 on C-2.

PATHOLOGIC FRACTURES OF THE SPINE

The vertebral column often is involved by a pathologic fracture inasmuch as it is a frequent site of bony metastasis, and on occasion the location of primary bone tumors. Most commonly, the body is involved in pathologic fractures, although the posterior arch may also be the site of fracture. The pedicles, however, are perhaps the most common site for early radiographic detection of bony metastasis to the spine. These fractures are described in routine fashion designating their location, the vertebrae involved, and noting the fact that the lesion is pathologic (Fig. II.93).

DISLOCATION OF THE SPINE

Dislocations of the spine occur when there is disruption of the supporting ligaments, leading to disruption of the posterior spinal joints and to loss of contact of the articular facets. Dislocation may involve one or both of the facet joints, leading to dislocation of a vertebra in part or as a whole, with rotary or lineal displacement. To be more specific, if one facet joint is dislocated, rotary displacement occurs, whereas, if both joints are dislocated, lineal displacement occurs (Fig. II.94). The cervical spine is most commonly involved. Dislocations of the spine are described by the direction of the displacement of the superior vertebra in relation to the inferior one. Most commonly, lineal dislocations occur in an anterior direction; however, posterior or lateral displacement may occur and be readily recognized. Rotary dislocation can occur in either direction (Fig. II.95).

Dislocation of the axis (C-1) may occur without fracture when there is rupture of the transverse atlantal ligament which runs posterior to the odontoid process. When this occurs, the stability of the C-1, C-2 articulation is lost and the atlas displaces anteriorly. The integrity of the spinal cord is severely jeopardized (Fig. II.96). This injury is described in the usual fashion by noting the displacement of the superior vertebrae, C-1, in relation to C-2.

FRACTURE DISLOCATION

Dislocations most frequently accompany fractures and result when there is disruption of the posterior bony elements. These fractures affect either the articular facets themselves or the pedicles, or, as in the case of the first and second cervical vertebrae, are associated with fracture of the odontoid. Fractures of these elements lead to loss of stability, resulting in displacement of the vertebra involved. Most commonly in these injuries, the superior vertebra is displaced anteriorly, with posterior dislocation being a rare injury. These injuries are designated as fracture dislocations, describing the resting position of the superior vertebra in relation to the one below and noting the section of the bone involved in the fracture.

Review

Identify the fractures illustrated (Figs. A–D). Correct identification is given on page 386.

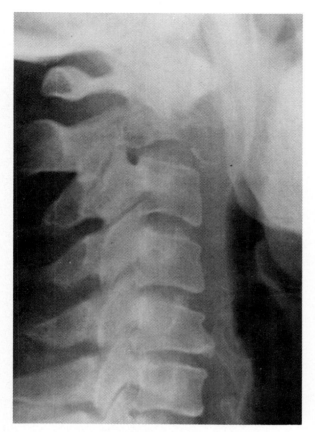

FIG. II.93. Pathologic compression fracture of the body of C-2.

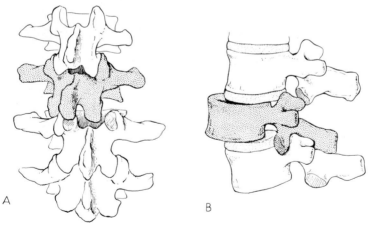

FIG. II.94. Dislocation of the spine may be due to involvement of one or both facets.

(A) Rotary displacement occurs when one facet is dislocated over another. Note the left inferior facet of the second vertebra is now lateral to the superior facet of the vertebra below. (After Watson-Jones.)

(B) Two facet joints have been dislocated, leading to lineal displacement anteriorly.

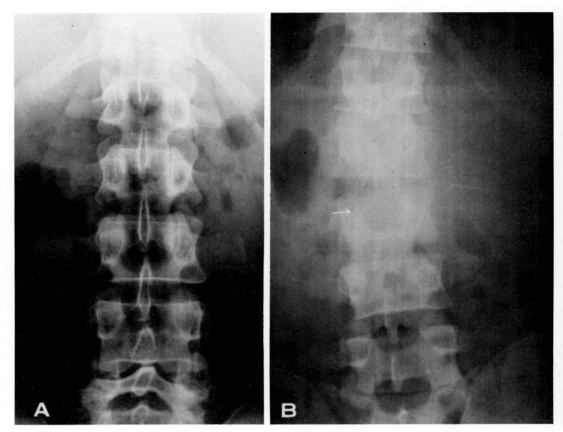

Fig. II.95.

(A) Normal anteroposterior roentgenograph of the lumbar spine. Note that the spinous processes are well aligned and that the superior facets of the vertebrae below are lateral to the inferior facets of the vertebrae above.

(B) Rotary displacement of L-2. Note that the spinous processes of L-3, 4, and 5 are no longer aligned with the upper ones and that the inferior facet of L-2 on the left lies outside of the superior facet of L-3.

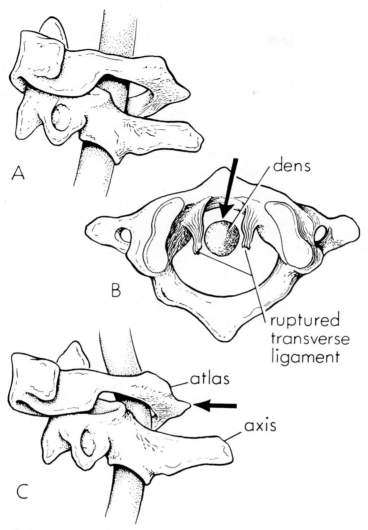

FIG. II.96. Rupture of the transverse ligament leads to forward subluxation of the axis.
  (A) Normal anatomic relationship of the atlas, axis, and spinal cord.
  (B) Overhead view showing rupture of the transverse ligament and loss of contact of the anterior arch of C-1 and odontoid.
  (C) Forward subluxation of C-1 on C-2, secondary to rupture of the transverse ligament. Note how the spinal cord can be compressed.

Figs. A–D.

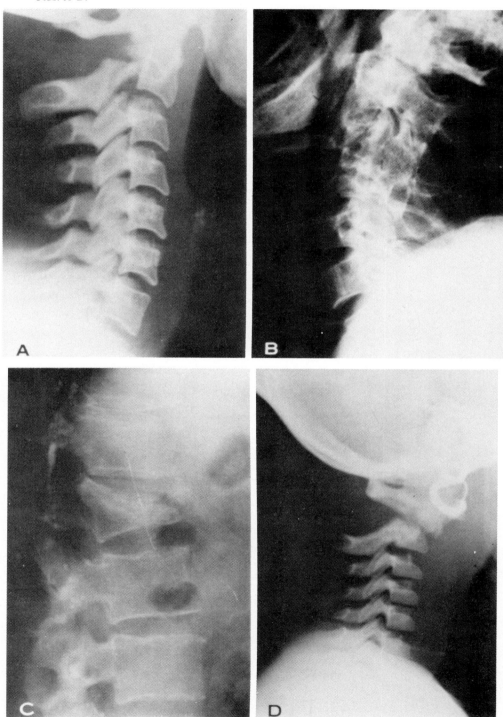

THE PELVIS

The bony pelvis is formed by the articulation of the two innominate bones and the sacrum which join each other to form a pelvic ring. The structure of these articulations is such that the innominate bones articulate with each other in front at the symphysis pubis, and with the sacrum posteriorly at the right and left sacroiliac joints (Fig. II.97).

The *innominate* bone is a large, irregularly shaped bone composed of three elements, the ilium, the ischium, and the pubis, which have a common point of junction in the region of the acetabulum. In childhood, during ossification, the three parts are distinct from one another and their junction at the acetabulum is cartilaginous and referred to as the triradiate cartilage.

The *ilium* (Fig. II.98) is the largest of the three elements and is an expanded segment of bone, somewhat in the shape of a fan. It consists of a body and a wing (ala), which are separated on the internal surface by the arcuate line, and on the outer surface by the margin of the acetabulum. The body is broad and forms approximately two-fifths of the acetabulum. The ala or wing is the large flared portion of the innominate bone, and has, in addition to its wide surfaces, a crest and several prominent tubercles. The iliac crest is the thickened superior border of the ilium. It exhibits an overhanging edge and its extent is marked by anterior and posterior bony projections, namely the anterosuperior and posterosuperior iliac spines. Ossification of the iliac crest is from a separate center than the ala and thus, prior to ossification, the crest is subject to avulsion fractures. Two other prominent tubercles are present, an anteroinferior iliac spine which serves for the origin of the direct head of the rectus femoris, and a posteroinferior iliac spine which is just superior to the greater sciatic notch.

The *ischium* is somewhat smaller than the ilium and is located at the posteroinferior aspect of the innominate bone (Fig. II.99). It is composed of four sections, a body, tuberosity, and two ischial rami. The body forms the posteroinferior aspect of the acetabulum and contains a posteromedial projection, the ischial spine. The greater sciatic notch,

185

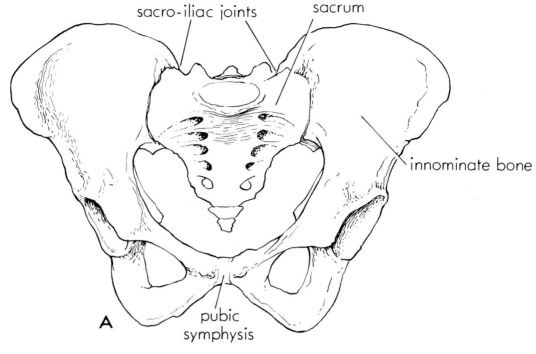

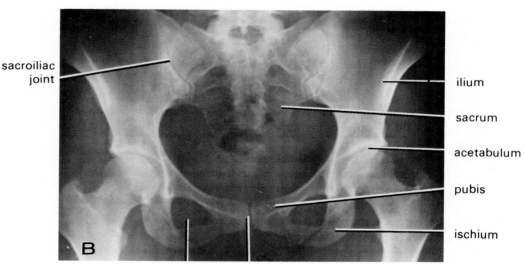

FIG. II.97.

(A) The bony pelvis is formed by the articulation of the two innominate bones and the sacrum to form a pelvic ring.

(B) Radiograph of the pelvic ring.

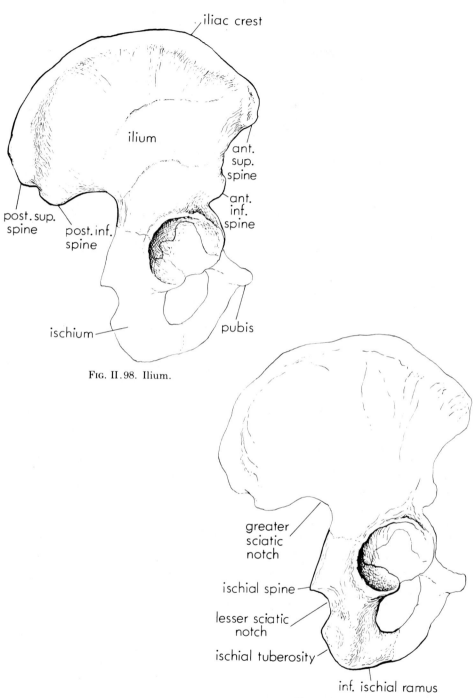

iliac crest

ilium

ant.
sup.
spine

ant.
inf.
spine

post. sup.
spine

post. inf.
spine

ischium

pubis

Fig. II.98. Ilium.

greater
sciatic
notch

ischial spine

lesser sciatic
notch

ischial tuberosity

inf. ischial ramus

Fig. II.99. Ischium.

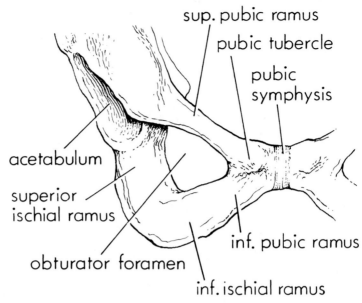

sup. pubic ramus

pubic tubercle

pubic symphysis

acetabulum

superior ischial ramus

obturator foramen

inf. pubic ramus

inf. ischial ramus

FIG. II.100. Pubis.

through which pass all the nerves of the gluteal region and posterior thigh, is located between the posteroinferior iliac spine and the ischial spine. Beneath the ischial spine is the lesser sciatic notch.

The inferior ischial ramus is a short flattened section of bone which projects somewhat anteriorly and joins the inferior ramus of the pubis.

The ischial tuberosity is a thickened area of bone and is the posterior projection of the superior ischial ramus. It lies between the body of the ischium and the ischial rami, and serves for the attachment of many strong muscles and ligaments, namely the adductor magnus muscle, sacrotuberous ligament, semimembranosus, long head of the biceps, and the semitendinosus muscle. When sitting, the body weight rests on the two ischial tuberosities.

The *pubis* (Fig. II.100 is composed of three parts, a body and a superior and inferior pubic rami. The body forms part of the acetabulum in conjunction with the body of the ilium and the body of the ischium.

The two pubic rami are relatively thin. Anteriorly, the superior ramus of the pubis joins its analogous mate, forming one of the articulations of the pelvis, the pubic symphysis. The inferior pubic ramus projects posterolaterally joining the inferior ischial ramus.

The *acetabulum* (Fig. II.101) is a cuplike cavity located at the lateral aspect of the innominate bone. It articulates with the head of the femur to form the hip joint. The rim of the acetabulum is prominent on its anterior, posterior, and superior aspects, thus providing bony stability

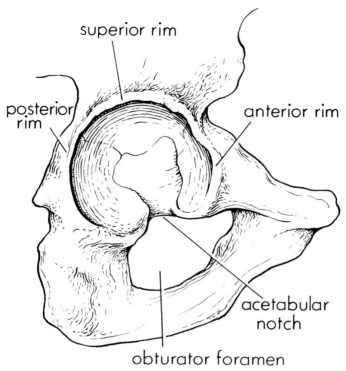

superior rim

posterior rim

anterior rim

acetabular notch

obturator foramen

FIG. II.101. Acetabulum.

for the hip joint. The superior aspect of the rim, in addition to contributing to stability, is the major weight-bearing portion of the acetabulum. Inferiorly, the acetabular rim is deficient, forming a deep notch called the acetabular notch.

Inferior to the acetabulum is a large somewhat circular orifice formed by encirclement of the bodies and rami of the ischium and pubis, known as the obturator foramen.

The pelvis is nearly a complete bony ring maintained by strong supporting ligamentous structures. The articulations of the bony pelvis include the sacroiliac joint and the symphysis pubis (Fig. II.97).

The sacroiliac joint is formed by the articulation of the articular surfaces of the sacrum and the ilium. These surfaces are covered with cartilage and are held together by the extremely strong sacroiliac ligaments.

The symphysis pubis is the anterior articulation of the pelvis and is formed by the junction of the medial aspect of the superior rami of the pubic bones. The articulating bony surfaces are covered with hyaline cartilage, separated by a fibrocartilaginous disc, and held together by the strong pubic ligaments.

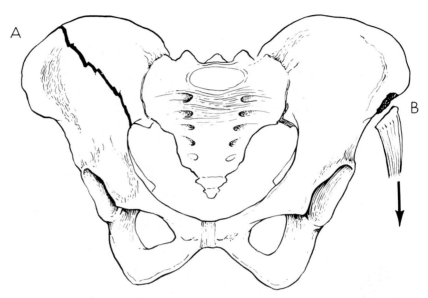

F<small>IG</small>. II.102. Fractures of the ilium.

(A) Oblique fracture through the wing of the ilium.

(B) Avulsion fracture of anteroinferior iliac spine.

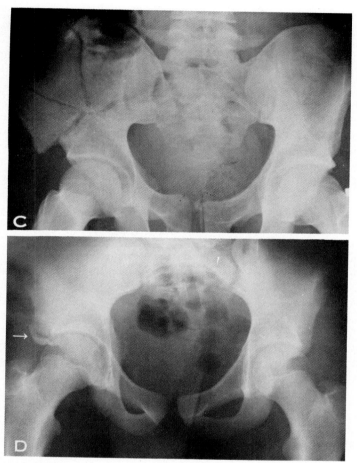

(C) Comminuted fracture of the wing of the left ilium. Note the stellate shape of the fracture lines.

(D) Avulsion fracture of the anteroinferior iliac spine on the left. The right side may be used for comparison.

INJURIES TO THE BONY PELVIS

Fractures of the pelvis are common and are usually the result of direct blows or crushing type injuries.

For descriptive purposes, fractures of the pelvis are considered to involve the basic anatomic structures, the pubis, ischium, ilium, acetabulum, and their articulations, namely the sacroiliac joint and the pubic symphysis. Fractures of the sacrum are not usually considered to be pelvic fractures.

Fractures of the pelvis are thus easily classified by noting the area of the pelvis involved and the nature and direction of the fracture; other descriptive terms are used as needed. It is not uncommon for multiple segments to be involved simultaneously, in which case each area can be described separately.

When assessing injuries to the bony pelvis, one must always be cognizant of the possibility of concomitant injury to the genitourinary tract and the abdominal viscera and, in addition, the possibility of massive amounts of retroperitoneal bleeding.

Fractures of the Ilium

Fractures of the ilium may be the result of direct trauma or avulsion forces. Fractures caused by direct trauma usually involve the wing or the crest of the ilium, whereas avulsion forces may involve the crest, especially in children. Most commonly, however, avulsion forces produce fractures of the anterosuperior and anteroinferior iliac spines. These fractures are simply described by the anatomic area involved, with further clarification made by noting the direction of the fracture, the presence of comminution, and if necessary, if an avulsion fracture has occurred (Fig. II.102).

Fractures of the Pubis

Fractures of the pubis are usually the result of direct trauma and may involve one or both rami. These injuries are simply described by the anatomic area involved, as the superior or inferior pubic rami, and, in addition, the direction of the fracture. Comminution and other descriptive terms may be applied (Fig. II.103).

Fractures of the Ischium

Fractures of the ischium may involve the ischial rami or the ischial tuberosities. As the ischium and pubis form a ring encircling the obturator foramina, a fracture through one section of the bony ring usually leads to fracture through another section. Thus fractures which involve the ischial rami usually occur in concert with fractures involving the pubic rami. As the line of anatomic demarkation is not always clear-cut on x-ray, it may be difficult to accurately differentiate fractures of the inferior ischial ramus from those of the inferior pubic ramus, unless

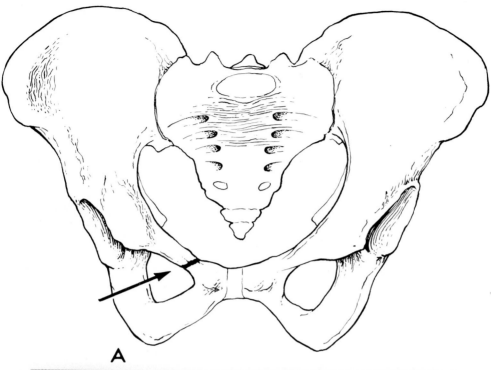

A

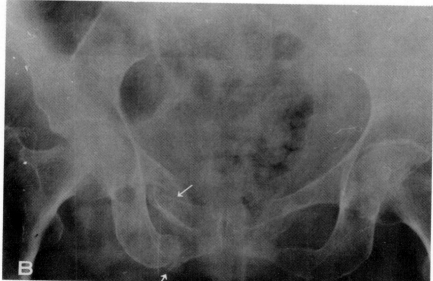

B

FIG. II.103. Fractures of the pubis.

(A) Diagram of an oblique fracture of the superior pubic ramus.

(B) Radiograph of a fracture of the superior and inferior pubic rami. Note the oblique fracture of the superior pubic ramus and a transverse fracture of the inferior pubic ramus.

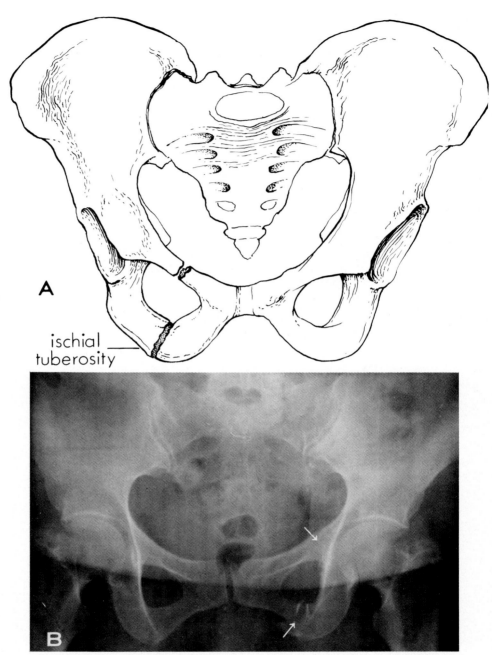

ischial
tuberosity

FIG. II.104. Fractures of the ischium.

(A) Diagram of transverse fractures of the inferior ischial ramus and superior pubic ramus.

(B) Comminuted fracture of the inferior ischial ramus associated with a transverse fracture of the superior pubic ramus. Since the rami form a ring, fracture through one area usually leads to fracture in another part of the ring.

the ischial ramus fracture is close to the ischial tuberosity. Fractures of the ischial rami are described by the location of the fracture and its direction and noting comminution, if present (Fig. II.104).

Fractures of the ischial tuberosity are usually caused by avulsion forces and are simply described as a fracture of the ischial tuberosity.

Fractures of the Acetabulum

Although the acetabulum forms part of the hip joint, fractures involving the acetabulum are commonly considered to be pelvic fractures.

Fractures of the acetabulum are usually caused by a force applied directly to the proximal femur (greater trochanter) or transmitted to it from a more distal site, driving the head of the femur against the acetabulum (see "Dashboard Fracture," page 301). As a result of this transmitted force, acetabular fractures may involve either the rim of the acetabulum or the central or medial aspect of the acetabulum. Commonly, dislocations of the hip accompany fractures of the acetabulum, although fracture may occur without dislocation.

Fractures of the acetabulum are described by the specific aspect of the acetabulum involved, such as the posterior, superior, or anterior rims (Fig. II.105). Fractures of the superior rim produce involvement of the weight-bearing component of the acetabulum and commonly result in a painful gait. Fractures of the posterior rim are commonly associated with instability of the hip, leading to recurrent subluxation or dislocation. Fractures which involve the medial aspect of the acetabulum are produced by a force which drives the head of the femur directly into the acetabulum, resulting in comminution of the acetabulum and displacement of the head of the femur into the pelvis. This injury is described as a central fracture dislocation of the hip (Fig. II.106) (see page 90).

Fracture Dislocations

Dislocations of the hip may complicate fractures of the acetabulum and are described by the area of the acetabulum involved and by the direction of the dislocation. The topic is discussed in the section on the hip (see page 96).

DISRUPTION OF THE ARTICULATIONS OF THE BONY PELVIS

As a result of trauma to the pelvis, there may be disruption of the articulations at either of the sacroiliac joints or symphysis pubis. Separation of these articulations is usually associated with fractures through the ring of the pelvis or by displacement of two articulations. This two site disruption occurs because the pelvis and its articulations form a ring, whereby wide separation and displacement at one joint in the ring requires distortion of the ring at another location. Thus this disturb-

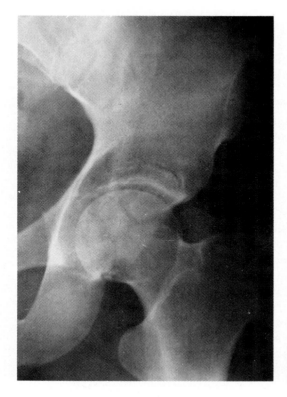

Fɪɢ. II.105. Comminuted fracture of the acetabulum. Note the comminution of the posterior rim with involvement of the superior rim.

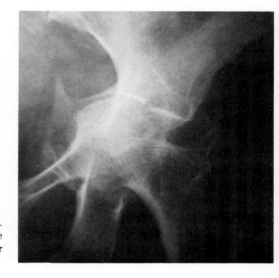

Fɪɢ. II.106. Central fracture dislocation of the hip. Note the marked comminution of the medial wall of the acetabulum, as well as some involvement of the superior rim.

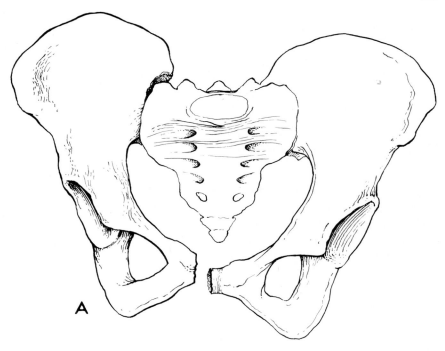

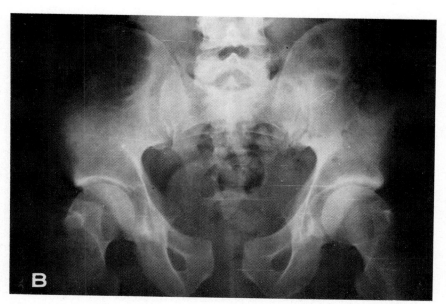

FIG. II.107 (A and B). Separation of the symphysis pubis and the sacroiliac joint. Displacement of one joint requires displacement of another, as the bony pelvis forms a ring.

ance may occur in any one of several patterns: (1) fracture through the bony pelvis at two locations, (2) fracture through the bony pelvis and disturbance of a single articulation, and (3) a disturbance of two articular surfaces (Fig. II.107).

Sacroiliac Joint

Disruption of the sacroiliac joint usually occurs by direct trauma, resulting in the ilium being displaced outward, upward, and posteriorly. This injury is designated as a dislocation of the sacroiliac joint (Fig. II.108).

Disruption of the Symphysis Pubis

Disruption of the symphysis pubis also occurs, usually as the result of direct trauma, and causes the articulating surfaces of the pubic symphysis to be separated. This may appear as a minimal displacement to a wide separation and is referred to as a separation of the pubic symphysis (Fig. II.109). With this injury, as with most pelvic injuries, one must always be alert to the possibility of concomitant injury of the genitourinary tract and the abdominal viscera.

Review

Identify the fractures illustrated (Figs. A–C). Correct identification is given on page 386.

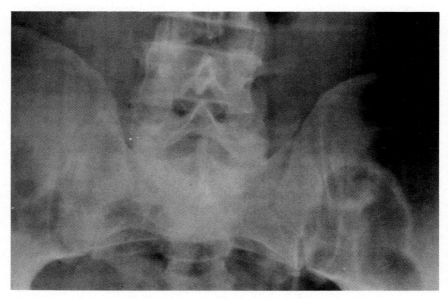

FIG. II.108. Separation of the right sacroiliac joint. Note the widening of the sacroiliac joint as compared to the opposite side.

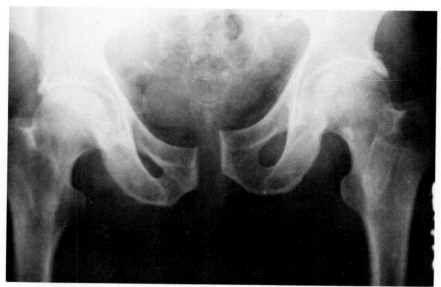

Fig. II.109. Separation of the pubic symphysis. Note the widening and the upward displacement of the pubis on the left.

Figs. A–C.

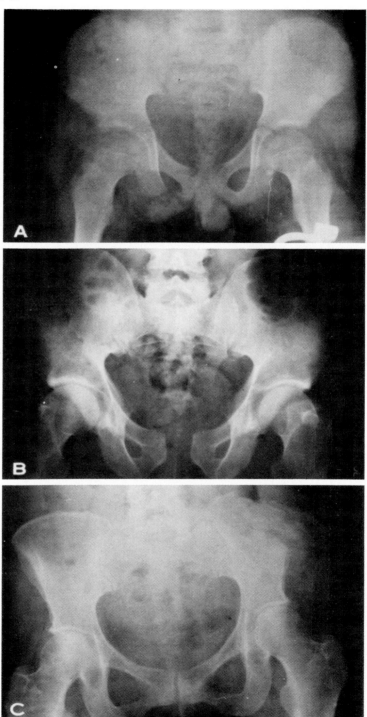

THE SHOULDER

The shoulder is the most movable and probably the least stable of all the joints of the extremities. Basically, it consists of the articulation of the glenoid fossa of the scapula with the head of the humerus (glenohumeral joint). When considering the mechanics of the shoulder with regard to injuries and motion, however, we must consider the articulations of the shoulder girdle to include the glenohumeral, the scapulothoracic, the acromioclavicular, and the sternoclavicular joints (Fig. II.110).

ANATOMY

Glenohumeral Joint (Shoulder Joint)

The glenohumeral joint (Fig. II.111) is a ball and socket joint possessing the greatest freedom of motion of all the joints of the body. Here, the large head of the humerus articulates with the shallow glenoid fossa of relatively smaller surface area.

The proximal aspect of the humerus bears some relation in configuration to the proximal aspect of the femur, inasmuch as there is a head, neck, two tuberosities, and a shaft.

The head of the humerus is smaller than that of the femur, being almost a hemisphere, and is directed medially upward and slightly backward. It is covered by articular cartilage and is joined to the shaft by a constricted area at the base of the head of the humerus called the anatomic neck. The anatomic neck is only a slight indentation at the base of the head into which the articular capsule attaches. Numerous vascular foramina perforate the anatomic neck. Located at the junction of the anatomic neck with the shaft of the humerus are the greater and lesser tuberosities, which afford attachment for the tendons of the rotator cuff muscles. The greater tuberosity is larger in size and projects laterally, whereas the lesser tuberosity projects anteriorly. The two tuberosities are divided by a groove, the intertubercular or bicipital sulcus, through which the tendon of the long head of the biceps runs.

A clinically important region, the surgical neck of the humerus lies just below the tuberosities or at the level where the tuberosities join the

201

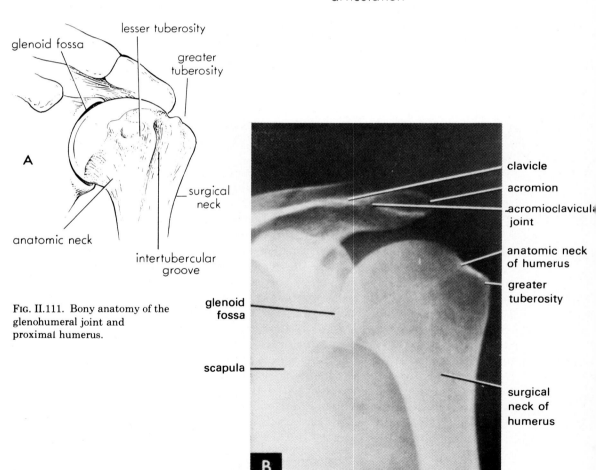

FIG. II.110. Articulations of the shoulder girdle include the glenohumeral, acromioclavicular, sternoclavicular, and scapulothoracic joints.

FIG. II.111. Bony anatomy of the glenohumeral joint and proximal humerus.

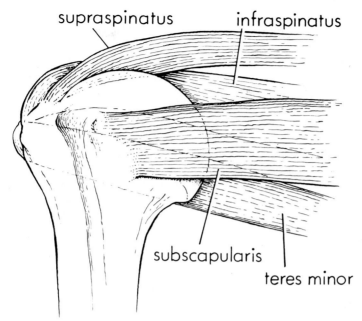

supraspinatus   infraspinatus

subscapularis

teres minor

FIG. II.112. Attachment of the rotator cuff muscles to the proximal humerus.

shaft of the humerus. On the medial aspect of the humerus, the surgical neck is contiguous with the anatomic neck.

The glenoid fossa is a shallow concavity located at the lateral angle of the scapula. It is somewhat oval in shape, covered with articular cartilage, and directed anteriorly and laterally. The glenoid fossa is deepened by the fibrocartilaginous glenoid labrum which is attached along the margin of the glenoid.

The fibrous capsule completely encircles the articular parts of the bones of the glenohumeral joint and is attached to the glenoid slightly proximal to the rim of the glenoid labrum, and distally inserts on the anatomic neck, medial to the two tuberosities. The capsule is relatively loose, and does not hold the bones of the joint in intimate contact, thus providing for the great freedom of motion that this joint possesses. The laxity can be demonstrated clinically in patients who have lost the function of the supporting muscles, for example, the deltoid muscle. In these cases, inferior subluxation of the head of the humerus occurs.

With the arm at the side or in adduction, the lower or medial aspect of the capsule is relaxed and lies in folds, becoming tense when the humerus is held in full abduction. The capsule is reinforced by the tendons of the short rotator cuff muscles and by various ligaments, namely the glenohumeral ligaments and coracohumeral ligament.

The strength and stability of the glenohumeral joint depends on the large muscles that pass over the joint and the four muscles which compose the rotator cuff, the supraspinatus above, the infraspinatus and teres minor behind, and the subscapularis in front (Fig. II.112). The tendons of the rotator cuff muscles blend intimately with the capsule and reinforce it. The rotator cuff muscles have the important function of retaining the head of the humerus in the socket and stabilizing it during motion of the shoulder.

The synovial membrane extends from the margin of the glenoid cavity and lines the inner surface of the capsule. It then reflects back onto the sides of the anatomic neck of the humerus up to the limits of the articular cartilage of the head.

As previously stated, shoulder motion is intimately concerned with the sternoclavicular, acromioclavicular, and the scapulothoracic joints, in addition to the glenohumeral joint, and a brief description of their anatomy will be presented.

Sternoclavicular Joint

The *sternoclavicular joint* (Fig. II.113) is a synovial joint formed by the articulation of the sternal end of the clavicle with the upper end of the sternum. An articular capsule surrounds the joint and is reinforced by anterior and posterior sternoclavicular ligaments. A fibrocartilaginous articular disc is interposed between the two articulating surfaces and possibly affords some stability and improves motion of the joint.

The sternoclavicular joint represents the only point of bony articulation between the trunk and upper limb. Thus the shoulder is virtually completely suspended by its muscles, ligaments, and capsule.

Acromioclavicular Joint

The *acromioclavicular joint* (Fig. II.114) is a synovial joint composed of an articulation between the lateral end of the clavicle and the acromion of the scapula. An articular capsule encloses the joint and is supported or reinforced by the acromioclavicular ligaments. A small articular disc is present, attached only to the superior aspect of the capsule.

The major stability of the acromioclavicular joint, however, is provided by the strong coracoclavicular ligament, anchoring the clavicle to the coracoid process of the scapula. This ligament consists of two parts, a trapezoid ligament and a conoid ligament. The conoid ligament is shaped like a cone with its apex pointed distally and is attached to the medial aspect of the coracoid process. The trapezoid ligament is situated anterolateral to the conoid ligament.

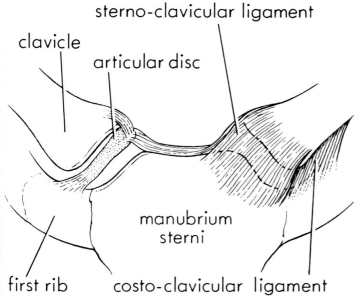

clavicle

sterno-clavicular ligament

articular disc

manubrium
sterni

first rib

costo-clavicular ligament

FIG. II.113. Sternoclavicular joint. The left side is a cross-sectional view demonstrating the articular disc. The right side shows the retaining ligaments.

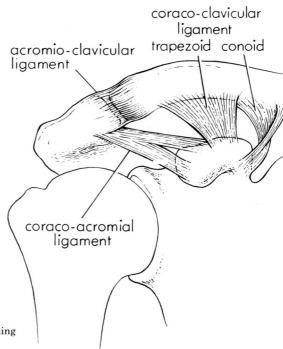

coraco-clavicular
ligament
trapezoid conoid

acromio-clavicular
ligament

coraco-acromial
ligament

FIG. II.114. Acromioclavicular joint and its retaining ligaments.

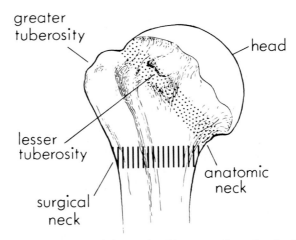

greater
tuberosity

head

lesser
tuberosity

anatomic
neck

surgical
neck

FIG. II.115. Anatomic structure of the proximal humerus allows for classification of fractures by area, namely the head, anatomic and surgical neck, and tuberosities.

Scapulothoracic Joint

The *scapulothoracic joint*, the articulation of the anterior surface of the scapula and the posterior rib cage, is not a true joint in that there is no apposition of bone to bone. Functionally speaking, however, in shoulder mechanics it behaves as a joint.

Restriction of motion at any of the four above junctions will restrict the total arc of motion of the shoulder.

Based on the descriptive anatomy of the proximal humerus, namely the head, anatomic neck, surgical neck, and tuberosities, and the various articulations concerned with shoulder motion and function, we have an arbitrary division which affords us a working vocabulary for the naming and description of shoulder injuries (Fig. II.115).

FRACTURES OF THE SHOULDER

The term, fracture of the shoulder, usually refers to those involving the proximal humerus, including the head, anatomic and surgical necks, and tuberosities.

Fracture Nomenclature

In the preceding paragraphs, we have established reference points based on anatomic location. Fractures occurring within these boundaries may now be classified:

1. Fracture of the neck of the humerus.
2. Fracture of the tuberosities.
3. Fracture of the humeral head.

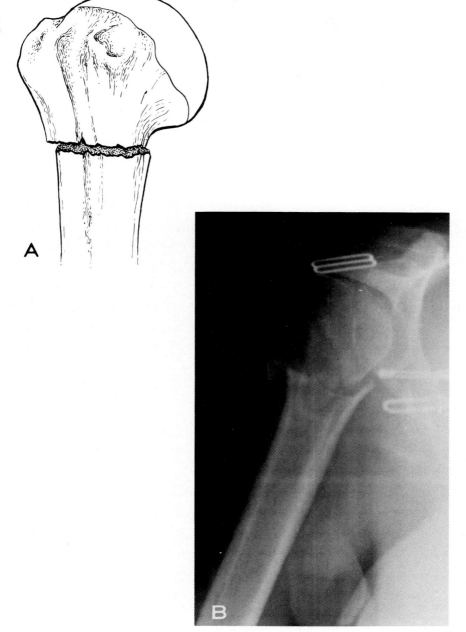

Fɪɢ. II.116. Fracture of the surgical neck of the humerus.
   (A) Diagram of transverse fracture.
   (B) Radiograph of a transverse fracture of the surgical neck.

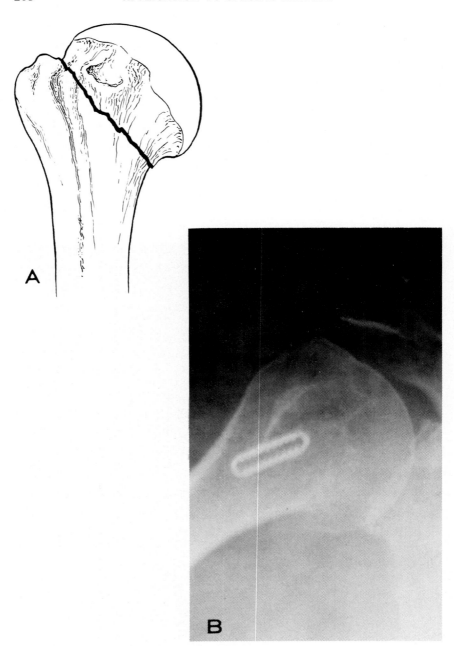

FIG. II.117. Fracture of the anatomic neck of the humerus.
  (A) Diagram of fracture.
  (B) Radiograph of a transverse fracture of the anatomic neck of the humerus. Note that there is some inferior displacement of the head.

Fracture of the Surgical and Anatomic Neck of the Humerus

Surgical Neck. Fracture of the *surgical neck* of the humerus is one of the most common types of shoulder fractures, and is a lesion that occurs just distal to the tuberosities, where the shaft of the proximal humerus is narrow (Fig. II.116). These fractures tend to be comminuted and may extend to involve the tuberosities and, at times, the anatomic neck of the humerus. Frequently, further descriptive classification of these fractures, as abduction and adduction fractures, is made, in relation to the position and alignment of the proximal and distal fragments. This classification will be discussed shortly.

Anatomic Neck. The *anatomic neck* is that short constricted section of bone just distal to the head of the humerus. Isolated fractures occurring through this level are rare and are referred to as fractures of the anatomic neck of the humerus (Fig. II.117).

Adduction and Abduction Fractures of the Neck of the Humerus

The normal head shaft angle of the proximal humerus is approximately 140°, and displaced fractures occurring in the region of the surgical neck tend to alter this angle. Frequently, displaced fractures of the neck of the humerus are described as abduction and adduction fractures, in a fashion similar to displaced fractures occurring in the neck of the femur. Unlike the hip, however, this assessment should be made judiciously, as depending upon the projection of the x-ray, the same fracture may show both adducted and abducted situations. Thus fractures may occur through the surgical neck and, depending on the rotational projection of the film, may appear to be in adduction or abduction (Fig. II.118).

In surgical neck fractures, however, rotation of the head may truly occur with the fracture assuming a position of adduction. At times, such severe rotation may occur that the articular margin of the head is in contact with the fracture surface of the distal fragment (Fig. II.119).

Fractures of the Greater and Lesser Tuberosities

Direct Trauma

Fractures of the greater tuberosity may be the result of direct trauma to the tuberosity or be an avulsion type, secondary to severe muscle contraction or dislocation of the shoulder. Fractures that occur as a result of direct trauma are usually comminuted and minimally displaced, and simply described by the anatomic area involved (Fig. II.120). Fractures of the lesser tuberosity are usually due to avulsion forces.

Avulsion Fractures

Avulsion fractures in the region of the shoulder occur at the greater

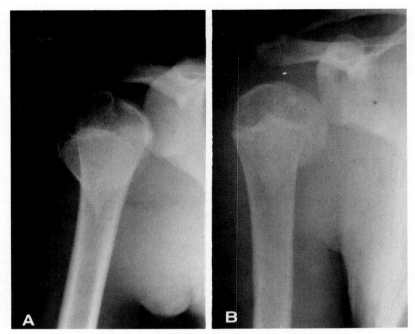

FIG. II.118 (A and B). Displaced fracture of the surgical neck. Note that in (A) the fracture appears to be in valgus or abduction, whereas in (B) the same fracture x-rayed in another projection appears now to be in varus or adduction.

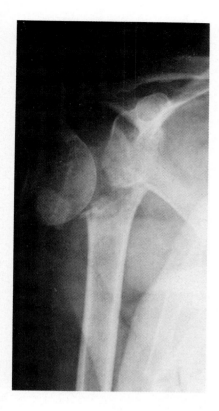

Fig. II.119. Transverse fracture of the surgical neck of the humerus with rotation of the head such that the articular surface of the head contacts the fracture surface of the distal fragment.

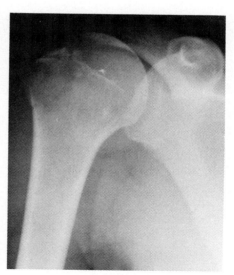

Fig. II.120. Comminuted fracture of the greater tuberosity. This fracture occurred as a result of direct trauma. Note the minimal separation and the comminution.

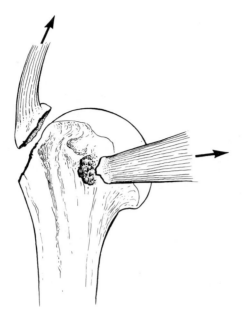

Fig. II.121. Avulsion fracture of the greater and lesser tuberosities. Note the forces of muscle contraction which produce the avulsion and distraction.

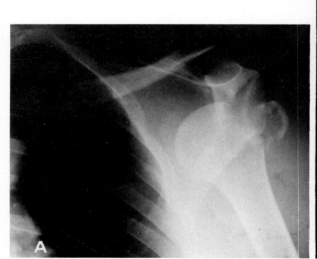
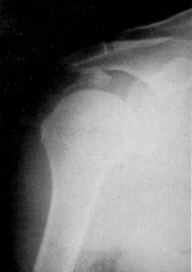

Fig. II.122.

(A) Avulsion fracture of the greater tuberosity associated with a dislocation of the head of the humerus.

(B) Avulsion fracture of the greater tuberosity with the fragment being pulled into position above the articular surface of the humerus.

and lesser tuberosities because of the attachments of the strong ligaments and muscles which make up the rotator cuff (Fig. II.121). The greater tuberosity serves for the insertion of the supraspinatous, infraspinatus and teres minor, and the lesser tuberosity for the insertion of the subscapularis muscle.

Separation of the greater tuberosity may occur as a result of forceful muscular contraction or by the rotator cuff muscles fixing the tuberosity in place when there is a dislocation of the head of the humerus.

In avulsion fractures, there is separation of the fracture fragments involving only that part of the tuberosity into which the tendon inserts. The separation may be minimally displaced, or so widely separated that the fragment of the greater tuberosity may retract into a position above the articular surface of the humerus (Fig. II.122).

Avulsion of the lesser tuberosity is a rare lesion and occurs as a result of forceful contraction of the subscapularis muscle. These fractures lend themselves to application of our routine terms and are designated as avulsion fractures of the greater or lesser tuberosity.

Fracture of the Humeral Head

Fractures of the humeral head are rare. When they do occur, they are usually associated with dislocation of the shoulder when, at the time of injury, a segment of the head is sheared off as the head strikes against the glenoid labrum. These fractures, designated as fractures of the head of the humerus, may also be considered as chondral or osteochondral fractures inasmuch as they are composed of a segment of articular cartilage or articular cartilage and bone (Fig. II.123).

Pathologic Fractures of the Shoulder

The proximal humerus is a frequent site for pathologic fractures of that bone. These fractures are usually the result of local disease such as primary bone tumors (benign and malignant), metastatic lesions, or at times, are due to radiation therapy. Pathologic fractures are usually located in the region of the surgical neck. These fractures are designated by their location and direction, with the additional information that they are pathologic.

DISLOCATION OF THE SHOULDER

Dislocation of the shoulder occurs when the head of the humerus separates from its normal articulation with the glenoid cavity of the scapula. Shoulder dislocations are probably the most common of all dislocations and may occur with or without associated fractures of either the head of the humerus, the tuberosities, or glenoid.

The designation of a shoulder dislocation is determined by the final resting position of the humeral head in relation to the glenoid cavity, and may be anterior, posterior, inferior, or superior.

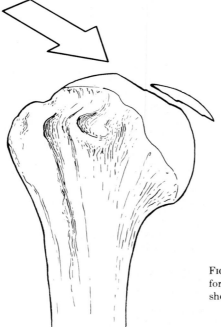

FIG. II.123. Fracture of the head of the humerus. The force arrow indicates that the fracture was due to a shearing blow.

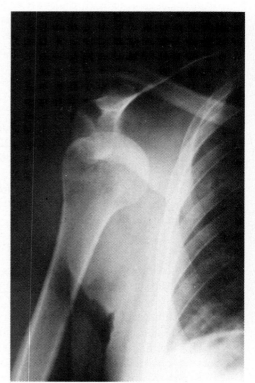

FIG. II.124. Anterior dislocation of the humerus.

Anterior Dislocations (Subcoracoid)

Anterior dislocations of the shoulder are the most common type and are ones in which the head of the humerus has come to rest anterior to the glenoid fossa. Inasmuch as this injury usually results in the head of the humerus lying beneath the coracoid process, it may also be referred to as a subcoracoid dislocation (Fig. II.124).

Posterior Dislocations

Posterior dislocations are less common and result when the head of the humerus lies posterior to the glenoid fossa. These injuries are difficult to interpret on routine anteroposterior radiographs and axillary or transthoracic views are necessary to confirm the diagnosis.

Infraglenoid Dislocations

This form of dislocation occurs when the head of the humerus comes to lie inferior to the glenoid (Fig. II.125). At times, with this type of dislocation, the arm is found fully elevated at the side of the patient's head—a position called luxatio erecta.

Superior Dislocation

This exceedingly rare lesion is one in which the head of the humerus comes to rest in front of the acromion.

Fracture Dislocations

Dislocations of the shoulder may occur in association with fractures, most commonly with fractures of the greater tuberosity (see Fig. II.122A).

Other areas that may be fractured, however, are the surgical neck and the head of the humerus, as well as the glenoid, the coracoid process, and the acromion (Fig. II.126). The description of these fracture dislocations should include the direction of the shoulder dislocation as well as a description of the accompanying fracture.

Recurrent Dislocation

Recurrrent dislocation of the shoulder is a common problem. With chronic dislocation, the head of the humerus and the glenoid are subjected to repeated injury and, as a result, two commonly reproducible lesions occur, the Hill-Sachs and the Bankhart lesions. The mechanism of injury that produces these lesions is the result of repeated anterior dislocations, such that with each episode the posterolateral aspect of the head of the humerus strikes against the anterior aspect of the glenoid.

The Hill-Sachs lesion is an osteochondral defect occurring on the posterolateral aspect of the head of the humerus, due to the repeated trauma. On x-ray projection, with the shoulder in internal rotation, the head of the humerus presents a hatchetlike appearance (Fig. II.127A).

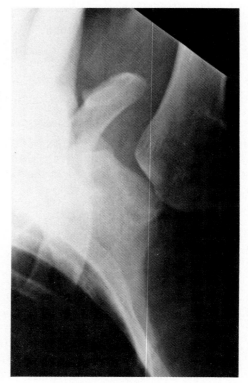

Fig. II.125. Infraglenoid dislocation. Note the arm extended in a position of luxatio erecta.

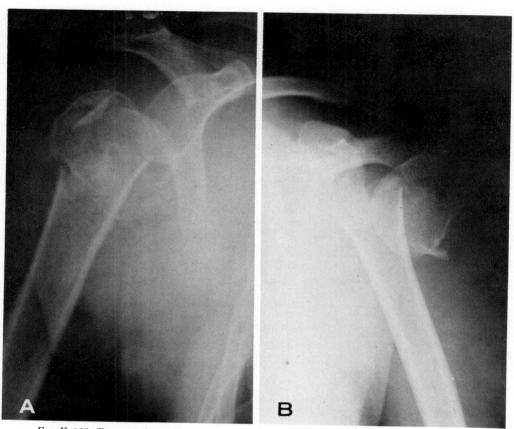

FIG. II.126. Fracture dislocations.

(A) Severe comminuted fracture dislocation of the head of the humerus with fracture through the surgical neck and comminution of the greater tuberosity.

(B) Transverse fracture of the surgical neck and dislocation of the head of the humerus.

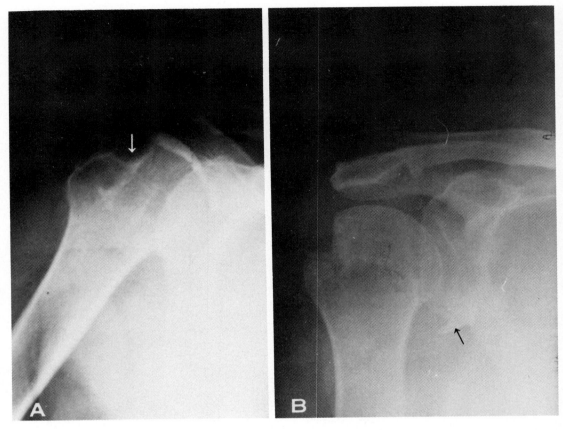

Fig. II.127.
(A) Hill-Sachs lesion. Note a hatchet deformity of the posterolateral aspect of the head of the humerus.
(B) Bankhart lesion occurring in association with a Hill-Sachs lesion. Note the fracture at the anteroinferior margin of the glenoid.

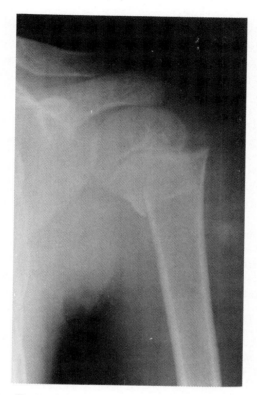

FIG. II.128. Separation of the proximal humeral epiphysis. Note that a fairly large fragment of metaphysis has accompanied the epiphyseal separation and thus it may be classified as a Salter-Harris Type II epiphyseal separation.

The Bankhart lesion is an injury to the anterior aspect of the glenoid which results in detachment of the labrum, or a chondral or osteochondral fracture of the anterior aspect of the glenoid. Radiographically, it can be demonstrated only if a bony fracture has occurred (Fig. II.127B).

INJURIES TO THE SHOULDER IN CHILDREN

The proximal humerus develops from three centers of ossification, one for the head and one for each tuberosity. At 5–8 years of age, these centers unite to form a single center. Separation of the proximal humeral epiphysis is probably the most common injury to the proximal humerus in children, usually resulting from indirect trauma applied to the elbow or outstretched hand. Isolated separation of the epiphysis is rare, the lesion usually containing a metaphyseal fragment. This injury is designated as an epiphyseal separation of the proximal humerus, and may be classified, if desired, by eponymic terminology, for example the Salter-Harris or Aitken classification (Fig. II.128). Avulsions of the epiphyses of the humerus also occur and are simply described by the epiphysis avulsed.

Epiphyseal separation and fractures through the surgical neck should not be confused with normal epiphyseal lines, which may readily occur because of the irregularity of the latter in older children (see Part IV, page 356). Comparative x-rays of the opposite shoulder are usually indicated in proximal humeral injuries.

Dislocation of the Proximal Humerus

Dislocation of the proximal humerus, although common in adults, is rare in children. This lesion is usually associated with pathologic changes in the proximal humerus, most commonly associated with nerve palsies. This lesion is named as a dislocation of the proximal humerus, or shoulder dislocation, and further described by the direction (Fig. II.129).

CLAVICLE

Anatomy

The clavicle is a long, doubly curved bone which serves as a prop to support the shoulder, and is the only bony attachment of the upper extremity to the thorax. In this position, it serves as a shock absorber, taking the brunt of forces transmitted through the outstretched arm to the shoulder or directly upon the shoulder. It is the first bone to ossify and is subcutaneous throughout its length. The clavicle articulates with the acromion at its lateral margin, forming the acromioclavicular joint and, with the sternum at its medial margin, forming the sternoclavicular joint (Fig. II.110, page 202).

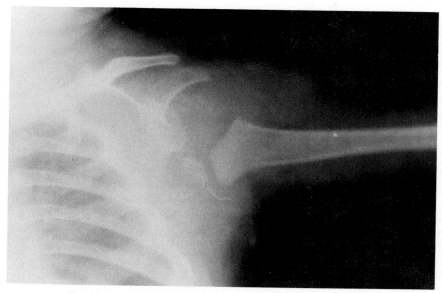

Fɪɢ. II.129. Infraglenoid dislocation of the shoulder in a child.

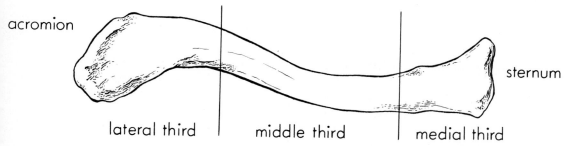

Fɪɢ. II.130. For reference, the clavicle may be divided into thirds, namely a medial or proximal, middle and lateral, or distal third.

Fracture Nomenclature

In consideration of injuries to the clavicle, we may divide the bone into a lateral, middle, and medial third (Fig. II.130). These segments have also been referred to as distal, middle, and proximal thirds. Fractures occurring in any of these regions may be designated in routine fashion as for any long bone, further modified by direction and comminution (Fig. II.131).

The articulation at either end of the clavicle, medially with the sternum and laterally with the acromion, presents two possible areas of dislocation and subluxation.

Acromioclavicular Joint Separation

Disruption of this joint is commonly referred to as a "shoulder separation." At the acromioclavicular joint, stability is achieved, in addition to the joint capsule, by two groups of ligaments, the acromioclavicular ligament and the coracoclavicular ligament, with the greatest amount of stability afforded by the latter (Fig. II.114, page 205).

Acromioclavicular Joint Subluxation

Acromioclavicular subluxation occurs if the acromioclavicular ligament and/or the capsule of the acromioclavicular joint is ruptured. As a result of the stability provided by the coracoclavicular ligaments, only slight displacement of the distal end of the clavicle in relation to the acromion occurs with some apposition of their articular surfaces remaining (Fig. II.132).

Acromioclavicular Joint Dislocation

Frank dislocation of the acromioclavicular joint occurs when both the acromioclavicular ligament and the coracoclavicular ligament are ruptured, resulting in complete separation of the clavicle and the acromion (Fig. II.133).

Acromioclavicular subluxations or dislocations, depending upon the magnitude of injury, may be associated with fractures of the clavicle.

Sternoclavicular Joint Dislocation

Disruption of the sternoclavicular joint is a rare injury and is referred to as sternoclavicular dislocation or subluxation. The displacement of the sternal border of the clavicle may be anterior, superior, or posterior, depending upon the forces which were responsible for the injury. The lesion is described as a sternoclavicular dislocation or subluxation and is named for the resting position of the medial border of the clavicle in relation to the sternum.

Review

Identify the fractures illustrated (Figs. A–E). Correct identification is given on page 386.

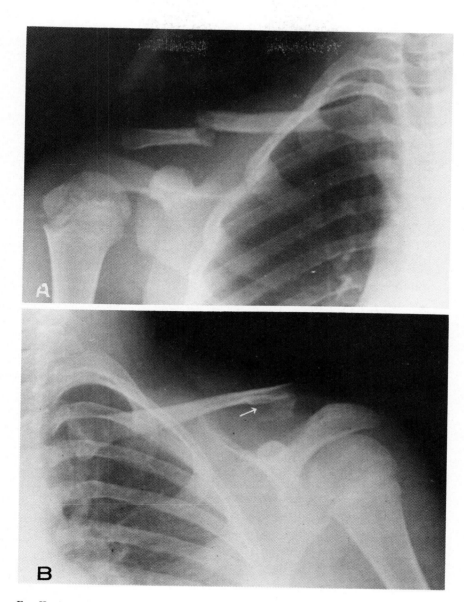

Fig. II.131.
    (A) Transverse fracture at the junction of the lateral and middle third of the clavicle.
    (B) Fracture of the distal third of the clavicle.

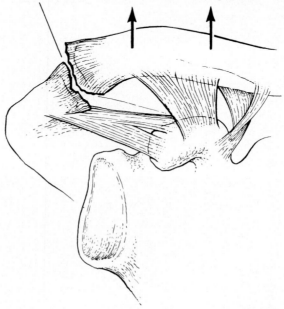

ruptured acromio-clavicular ligament

FIG. II.132. Acromioclavicular subluxation. Note that only the acromioclavicular ligament is ruptured and that there is slight displacement with some apposition of the articular surfaces of the acromion and the clavicle.

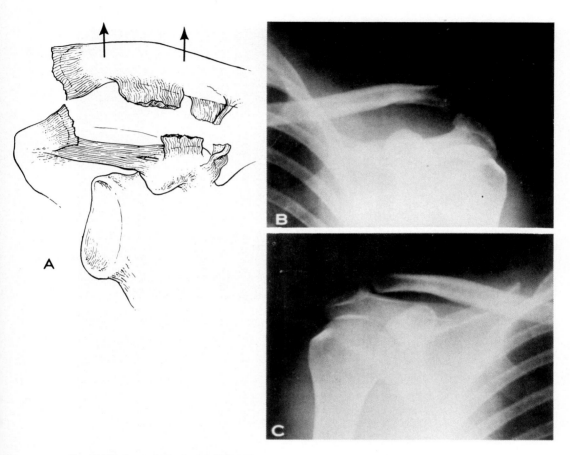

Fɪɢ. II.133. Acromioclavicular dislocation.

(A) In this injury, the acromioclavicular and the coracoclavicular ligaments are ruptured and there is loss of contact between the acromion and the clavicle.

(B) Radiograph of acromioclavicular dislocation. Note the high riding position of the clavicle.

(C) Comparative view of the opposite shoulder.

Figs. A–B.

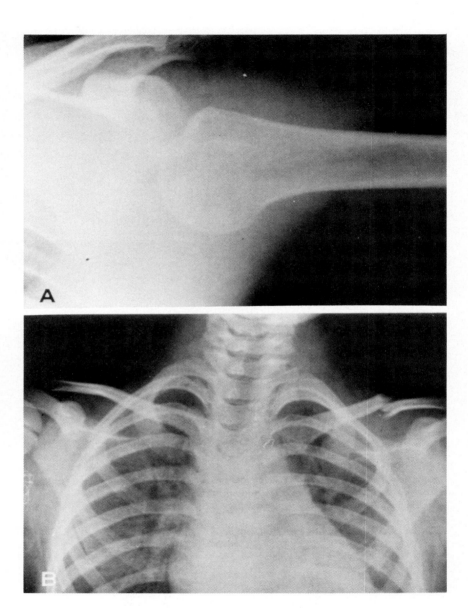

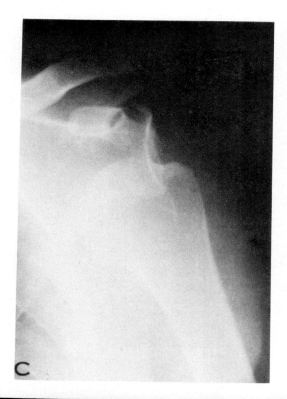

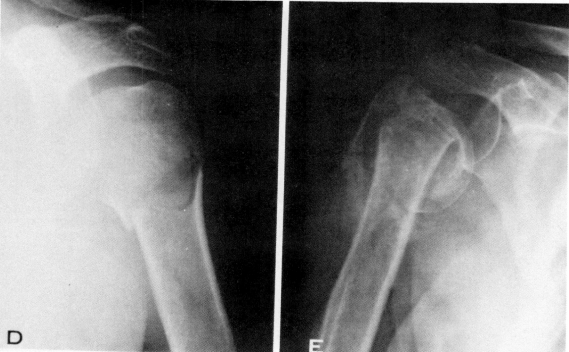

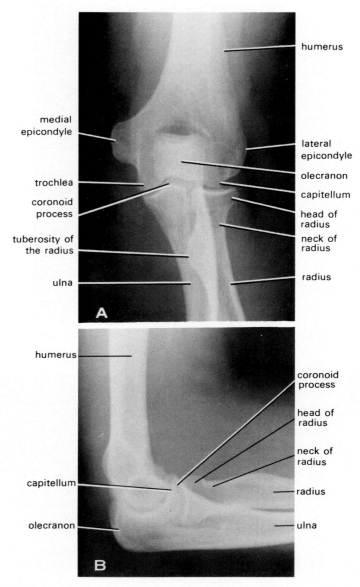

Fig. II.134 (A and B). Anteroposterior (A) and lateral (B) radiograph of the normal elbow. Note the anterior tilt of the humeral condyles.

THE ELBOW

ANATOMY

The elbow is a synovial joint formed by the articulation of the distal humerus with the proximal ulna and radius, forming a humeroulnar and humeroradial articulation. In addition, there is a junction of the head of the radius with the ulna forming a proximal radioulnar articulation (Figs. II.134 and II.135).

The humeroulnar articulation, a hinge or ginglymus joint, allows for uniaxial motion perpendicular to the long axis of the bones, articulating the spool-shaped trochlea of the medial aspect of the distal humerus with the concave trochlear notch of the ulna. The radiohumeral articulation also allows for uniaxial motion, however, in a different plane, being a pivot or trochoid joint, articulating the spherical capitellum with the cup-shaped surface of the head of the radius (Fig. II.135).

Distal Humerus (Figs. II.134 and II.136)

The distal humerus expands into a somewhat flattened and bulbous structure formed by the humeral condyles, and is further widened by two projections, the medial and lateral epicondyles, which are continuous with the supracondylar ridges of the humerus and lie just superior to the articular end of the humerus. The medial epicondyle forms a large prominence on the medial aspect of the elbow, whereas the lateral epicondyle is considerably shorter. The epicondyles serve for tendon attachments, with the flexor pronator group of muscles arising from the medial epicondyle and the extensor group from the lateral epicondyle.

The distal articular surface of the humerus is a continuation of the condyles and is divided into two sections; the spool-shaped trochlea, comprising the medial section, and the globular capitellum, forming the lateral aspect of the articular margin. These regions will articulate with the trochlear notch of the ulna and cup-shaped head of the radius, respectively. When viewed from the side, the condyles and articular processes tilt anteriorly approximately 45° (Fig. II.134).

Two major depressions are present just superior to the trochlea, the

229

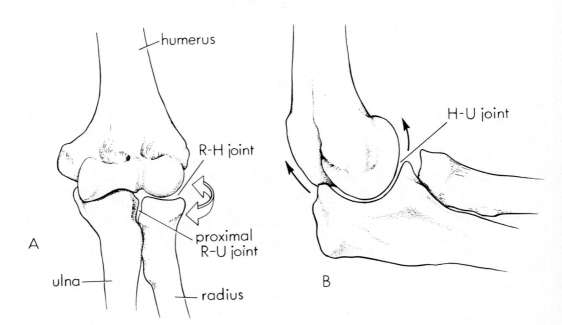

Fig. II.135 (A and B). Articulations of the elbow are formed by the distal humerus with the proximal ulna and radius (humeroulnar and humeroradial articulation), and the head of the radius with the ulna (proximal radioulnar articulation). Uniaxial motion occurs in two planes: (A) The trochoid motion of the radiohumeral joint and, (B) the ginglymus action of the humeroulnar articulation.

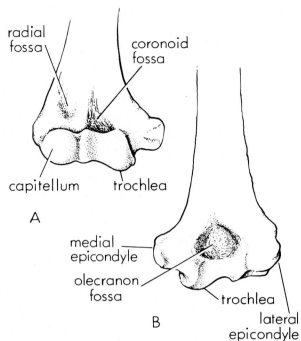

FIG. II.136 (A and B). Distal humerus.
Anterior view (A), posterior view (B).

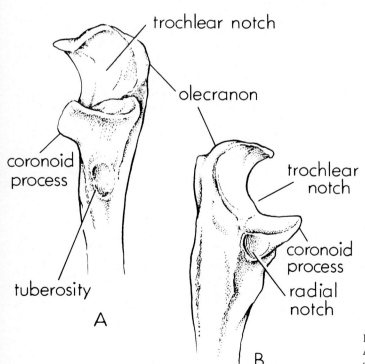

FIG. II.137 (A and B). Proximal ulna.
Anterior view (A), and from the radial
side (B).

olecranon fossa posteriorly which will receive the olecranon of the ulna in extension, and the coronoid fossa anteriorly which will receive the coronoid process of the ulna in flexion. There is also a minor depression anteriorly to receive the head of the radius in flexion, the radial fossa.

Proximal Ulna (Figs. II.134 and II.137)

The proximal ulna is a thickened area of bone which is deeply grooved on its anterior surface, forming the concave trochlear notch. Posterior to the trochlear notch is the olecranon, a thick buttress of bone which forms the posterior projection of the elbow. At the anterior margin, the trochlear notch ends in a triangular projection, the coronoid process, which serves for the insertion of the brachialis muscle. To receive the head of the radius, there is a shallow concavity on the lateral side of the coronoid process called the radial notch.

Proximal Radius

The proximal radius (Figs. II.134 and II.138) consists primarily of two main descriptive sections, a head and neck. The head of the radius is a disc-like articular surface in the form of a shallow cup which articulates with the capitellum of the humerus. Just beneath the head is a constricted area of bone, the neck of the radius, which ends at the radial tuberosity. The latter serves as the attachment for the biceps tendon.

A fibrous capsule encloses and adds stability to the articulation of the elbow. The capsule is attached anteriorly to the humerus, extending from the medial and lateral epicondyles along the coronoid and radial fossae, and inserts distally into the anterior border of the coronoid process of the ulna and the annular ligament of the radius. The capsule is strengthened by the collateral ligaments which are present on the medial and lateral aspects of the joint and are taut in all degrees of flexion and extension. The head of the radius is held in position by the annular ligament which is attached to the ends of the radial notch of the ulna.

The synovial membrane of the elbow lines the capsule and is present in redundant folds, thus permitting flexion-extension and rotary motion of the elbow.

INJURIES TO THE ELBOW

Bony injuries in the region of the elbow may involve the distal end of the humerus, the proximal end of the ulna, and the proximal end of the radius, and may be described simply, if we apply our general fracture terms to the anatomic structures of the elbow. Thus we may use the established reference points and describe the injuries of the elbow as occurring at:

1. The distal humerus.
2. The proximal ulna.

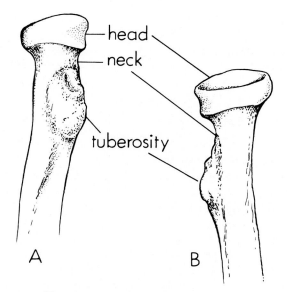

Fig. II.138 (A and B). Proximal radius.

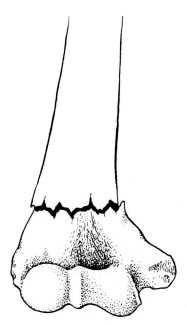

Fig. II.139. Supracondylar fractures are fractures which occur above the level of the condyles.

3. The proximal radius.
4. The humeroulnar articulation.
5. The humeroradial articulation.
Fractures occurring within these boundaries may now be classified.

Distal Humerus

Fractures of the distal humerus are described in relation to the humeral condyles, the epicondyles, the trochlea, and the capitellum.

Fractures Related to the Condyles

Supracondylar Fractures. Supracondylar fractures of the humerus are the most common elbow fractures in children and adolescents, and are fractures occurring above the humeral condyles (Fig. II.139).

The fracture is named for its anatomical location and further described as to direction, nature of injury, and type of displacement. The latter, described by the position of the distal fragment in relation to the proximal one, is usually posterior. In addition, the distal fragment may be displaced either laterally or medially with a rotary component (Fig. II.140).

Intercondylar Fractures. Fractures passing through the level of the condyles of the humerus are considered intercondylar fractures or transcondylar fractures. Intercondylar fractures occur in various patterns, depending upon the direction and comminution of the fracture. A single fracture line may be present and involve one or both condyles in transverse, oblique, or more vertical patterns. These fractures are named for the condyle involved and the direction of the fracture (Fig. II.141). A transverse fracture extending through both condyles is referred to as a transcondylar fracture (Fig. II.142).

In addition, comminuted fractures may occur, some with multiple fragments and fracture lines running in many different directions, and others in which a pattern may be formed by the fracture line. These are described by the pattern formed, the most common patterns being those of T or Y fractures (Fig. II.143). These fractures usually extend into the joint and, therefore, are intraarticular in nature.

Fractures of the Capitellum

A fracture of the capitellum usually occurs as the result of a valgus injury to the elbow, causing the head of the radius to be driven upward and forward delivering a shearing blow to the front of the capitellum. The head or neck of the radius may also be fractured but most commonly is not (Fig. II.144). The fracture line is readily visible on the anterioposterior radiograph; however, it may be difficult to interpret on the lateral projection. If viewed from the lateral aspect, the capitellum is located anterior to the long axis of the humerus, forming an angle of

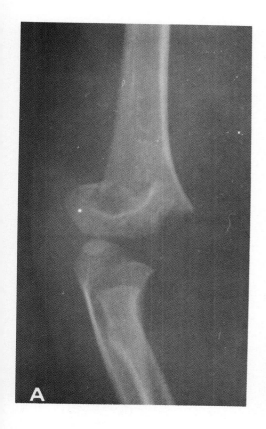

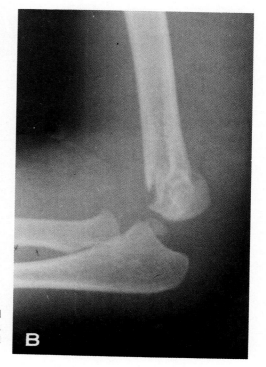

Fig. II.140 (A and B). Anteroposterior (A) and lateral (B) radiograph of a transverse supracondylar fracture. Note that the distal fragment is rotated and displaced posteriorly and medially.

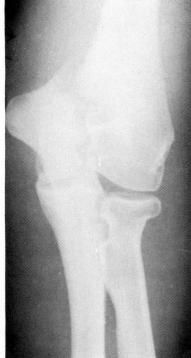

Fig. II.141. Vertical intercondylar fracture separating the medial condyle and extending into the joint.

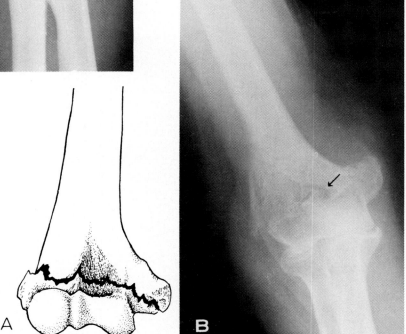

Fig. II.142. Transcondylar fracture.

(A) Diagrammatic representation. Note that the fracture extends through both condyles.

(B) Roentgenograph of transcondylar fracture.

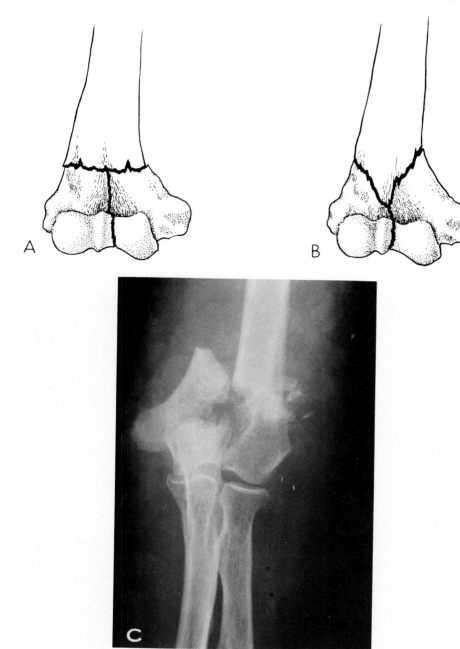

FIG. II.143. Comminuted intraarticular fractures of the distal humerus.
  (A) T-shaped fracture.
  (B) Y-shaped fracture.
  (C) Radiograph of a T-shaped fracture.

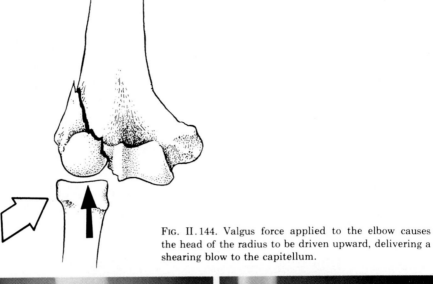

FIG. II.144. Valgus force applied to the elbow causes the head of the radius to be driven upward, delivering a shearing blow to the capitellum.

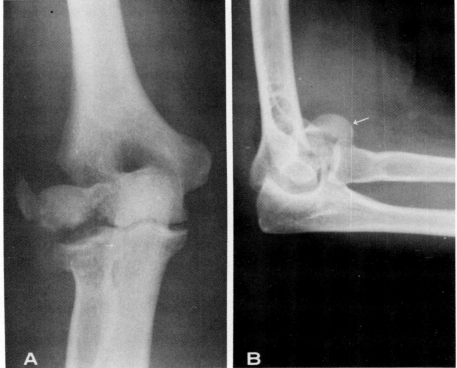

FIG. II.145 (A and B). Anteroposterior (A) and lateral (B) roentgenograph of a fracture of the capitellum. Note the rotation of the fragment and that the articular surface is facing upward. There is an accompanying fracture of the head of the radius.

approximately 45° with the shaft. Alteration of this angle occurs with displacement of the capitellum fragment. This displacement is usually in an anterior direction (Fig. II.145).

Fractures of the capitellum are named for their anatomical location and further described by the final position of the displaced fragment.

As the capitellum is continuous with the lateral condyle, fractures involving the capitellum may also involve the lateral condyle. These injuries are considered fractures of the lateral condyle and classified as such. Fractures involving the condyles and epicondyles will be discussed further under children's fractures about the elbow.

Proximal Ulna

Fractures of the proximal ulna are also described by the anatomic area involved, with basically two sites to be considered, the olecranon and the coronoid process (Fig. II.146).

The *olecranon*, because of its superficial position and attachment to a strong tendon and muscle mechanism, is much like the patella in being subject to both direct and indirect trauma. Any fracture extending into this area, despite the size of the fragment, is described as a fracture of the olecranon. Because of the attachment and strong pull of the triceps muscle, complete fractures through the olecranon are usually distracted, despite the mechanism of injury. These fractures are further described by the direction of the fracture line, the amount of comminution, and the presence or absence of displacement (Fig. II.147).

The *coronoid process* is the bony insertion of the brachialis muscle, and the fractures are usually of the avulsion variety. These fractures are simply described by the area involved (Fig. II.148).

Proximal Radius

The radius may be fractured in either the region of the head or neck. These fractures usually occur with a valgus injury to the elbow and are produced by impaction of the radial head by the capitellum of the humerus, the mechanism of injury being similar to depression fractures of the tibial plateaus at the level of the knee. The result of this injury is either angulation at the neck or fragmentation of the head of the radius (Fig. II.149). A fracture of the capitellum, at times, can accompany the fracture of the radius.

Fractures of the Head of the Radius

Fractures of the head of the radius occur either at the rim of the articular margin, adjacent to, or more commonly, at a distance from the proximal radioulnar joint, or involve the entire articular surface of the head of the radius. All varieties of this injury occur, ranging from single linear fractures to severe comminution. The fractures are designated as fractures of the head of the radius and are further described by the

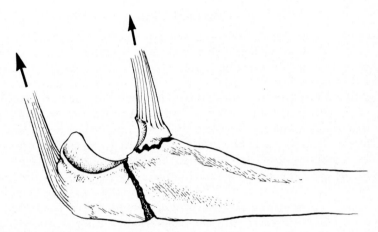

Fig. II.146. Fracture of the olecranon and coronoid process. Muscle contraction can cause distraction of fracture fragments.

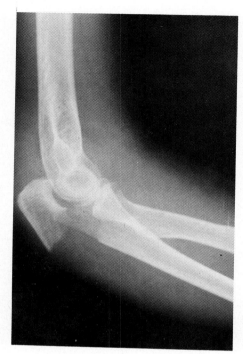

FIG. II.147. Closed fracture of the olecranon. Note the distraction and the somewhat transverse nature of the major fracture line.

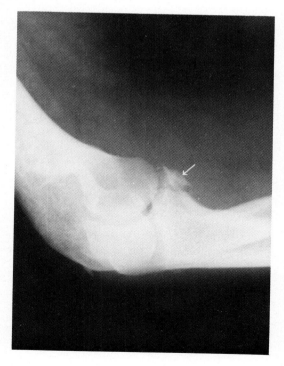

FIG. II.148. Fracture of the coronoid process. Note that the fragment is avulsed slightly upward.

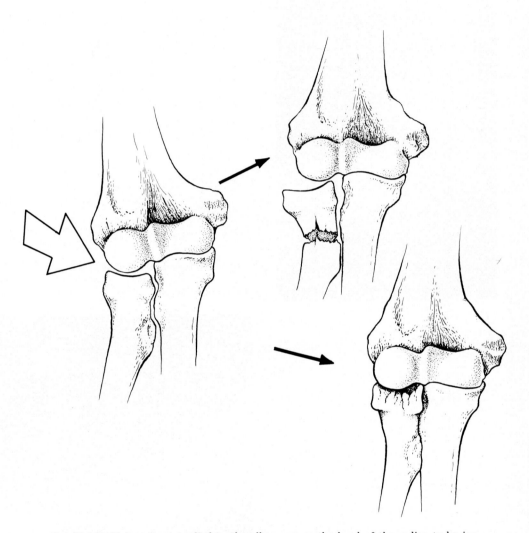

Fig. II.149. Valgus force applied to the elbow causes the head of the radius to be impalled against the capitellum and produce either a fracture of the head or neck of the radius.

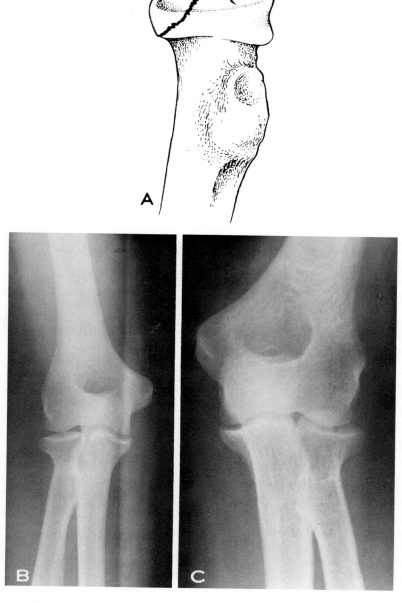

Fig. II.150. Fractures of the head of the radius.
   (A) Diagram of a comminuted fracture of the head of the radius.
   (B) Linear nondisplaced fracture of the head of the radius.
   (C) Fracture of the outer rim with inferior and lateral displacement.

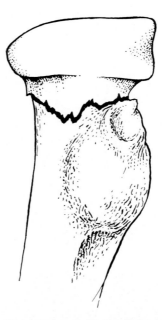

Fɪɢ. II.151. Transverse nondisplaced fracture of the
neck of the radius.

amount of the head involved and the comminution, displacement, and
angulation of the rim (Fig. II.150).

Fractures of the Neck of the Radius

Fractures occurring below the level of the head are simply described
as fractures of the neck of the radius. Fractures of the neck of the radius are named for their anatomical location, the direction of the fracture, and the angulation that is produced (Fig. II.151).

Avulsion Fractures of the Elbow

The elbow is a prime site for avulsion fractures, especially in children, as the bony prominences serve for the origins or insertions of
many strong muscles. Avulsion fractures of the humerus occur either at
the lateral or medial epicondyle, whereas those of the ulna occur at the
olecranon and the coronoid process. Avulsion fractures of the radius
occur at the radial tuberosity. These fractures are described as avulsion fractures of the area involved and further elaborated on by the
direction of the fracture and the degree of displacement.

Fractures of the Elbow in Children

The elbow is a common site of injury in children, and because of the
complexities associated with difficulty in diagnosis, and frequency of
complications, this subject requires special attention.

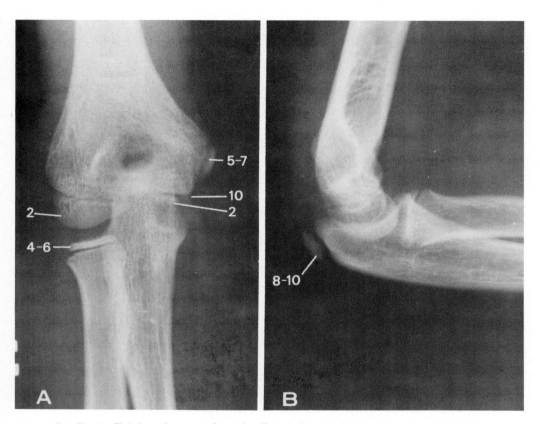

FIG. II.152. Epiphyseal centers about the elbow indicating the age of ossification in years. Note the lateral epicondyle is not yet ossified and the early ossification of the medial aspect of the trochlear.

The distal humerus and proximal ulna and radius ossify from several centers which appear at different times of life. There are epiphyseal centers for the trochlea, capitellum, lateral epicondyle, and medial epicondyle of the humerus (the trochlea having a double center), as well as a center of ossification for the head of the radius and the olecranon of the ulna. The appearance of these centers occurs in the following order which is quite consistent for a specific age.

Ossification of the capitellum and lateral aspect of the trochlea appears at 2 years of age, whereas the medial epicondyle appears at 5–7 years of age. Ossification of the other components of the distal humerus include the medial aspect of the trochlea which appears at 10 years of age and the lateral epicondyle at 10–12 years of age. The head of the radius begins to ossify at 4–6 years of age and the olecranon at 8–10 years of age (Fig. II.152).

It is of somewhat more than academic interest to know the age at which ossification occurs, as displacement of the epiphysis in injury may be recognized by identifying the individual ossification centers and noting their relationship to the parent bone. The diagnosis of injury to an unossified area may be based only on clinical evidence. Secondly, misinterpretation of fractures on x-ray may occur if the age of ossification is not known by mistaking an epiphysis for an avulsion fracture or a fracture line as an epiphyseal plate. Comparative x-rays may assist in the diagnosis and should be taken in all elbow injuries in children and adolescents.

Supracondylar Fractures in Children

A supracondylar fracture is one of the most common fractures of the elbow in children and is produced by a fall on the hand with the force being transmitted through the partially flexed forearm bones to the elbow. The distal fragment is most commonly displaced medially and posteriorly, and rotation is usually present (Fig. II.140, page 235).

Supracondylar fractures are probably fraught with more complications than any other fracture in children, and include malunion, tardy ulnar nerve palsy, and circulatory compromise.

Complications of Supracondylar Fractures

1. Malunion—cubitus valgus and varus.
2. Tardy ulnar nerve palsy.
3. Circulatory compromise.

Malunion. When treating supracondylar fractures of the humerus, difficulty is frequently experienced in obtaining anatomic reduction even in the most experienced hands, and resulting malunion is not uncommon. This malunion usually manifests itself in valgus or varus malalignment at the elbow.

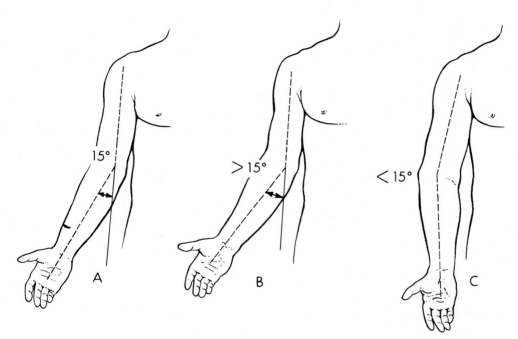

Fig. II.153. Deformities occurring as a result of malunion of a supracondylar fracture of the elbow.

(A) Normal carrying angle of the elbow with approximately 15° of valgus.

(B) Cubitus valgus—an increase laterally of the normal carrying angle.

(C) Cubitus varus—the normal carrying angle is reversed with the forearm assuming a position of medial displacement.

Cubitus Valgus and Varus. With the hands placed at the sides in the normal anatomic position, that is, with the palms forward and elbows extended, the forearm, in relation to the upper arm, is maintained at an angle of approximately 15–20° of valgus. This angle is known as the carrying angle (Fig. II.153). *Cubitus valgus* is a deformity of the elbow occurring when there is an increase laterally in the carrying angle.

Cubitus varus is an elbow deformity occurring when there is a decrease or reversal of the carrying angle with the forearm assuming a position of medial displacement. This reversal of the carrying angle produces a common clinical deformity of the elbow known as a gunstock deformity.

The terms cubitus valgus or varus are not reserved just for fractures but are applied to any situation where there is an alteration of the normal carrying angle. Improper reduction of fractures with a resultant malunion is probably the most common cause; however, asymmetric epiphyseal growth secondary to congenital malformation or infection, as well as trauma, produce deformities which alter the normal carrying angle and result in cubitus valgus or varus.

Tardy Nerve Palsy. Cubitus valgus places undue traction on the ulnar nerve which passes along the medial aspect of the elbow. As a result of the increased stretch placed on the nerve, patients may have resultant nerve palsies secondary to this position, some of which may first become clinically evident many years after injury.

Circulatory Compromise. Probably the most drastic complication of a supracondylar fracture is that of circulatory compromise with resultant Volkmann's ischemic contracture. The pathology is the result of interruption of the normal circulation to the forearm due to involvement of the brachial artery. The arterial occlusion may be the result of laceration of the artery, arterial spasm and reflex spasm of the collateral circulation, entrapment of the artery between the fracture fragments following reduction, or, as most commonly occurs, is secondary to severe tense swelling in the region of the elbow which subsequently impedes the circulation. As a result, there is direct effect on the flexor muscles and nerves of the forearm, leading to ischemic muscle and nerve changes with resultant flexion contractures of the hand and wrist and impairment of sensation.

Epiphyseal Injuries

Following supracondylar fractures, epiphyseal injuries are the commonest of bony injuries about the elbow in children. The multiplicity of epiphyseal centers, some of which are traction epiphyses and some pressure epiphyses, predispose the elbow to many varieties of epiphyseal injuries of both direct trauma and avulsion forces. As the cartilaginous epiphyseal line is a potential zone of weakness, it will tend to

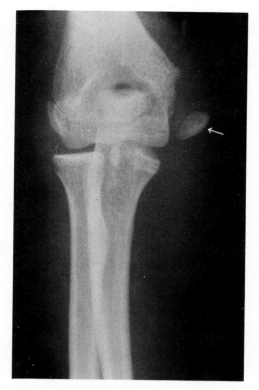

FIG. II.154. Avulsion fracture of the medial epicondyle of the elbow. Note that the fragment is rotated
and displaced downward due to the pull of the flexor
pronator group of muscles which arise from this area.

separate first as opposed to ligament rupture or fracture of the adjacent
bone. A fall on the flexed elbow may displace the entire distal humeral
epiphysis forward, whereas a valgus stress to the elbow may cause the
epiphysis of the medial epicondyle to be avulsed by the common flexor
group of muscles, and similarly when the joint is forced into varus, the
lateral epicondyle may be avulsed by the common extensor muscles.

The epiphyseal injuries at the elbow, therefore, include displacement
of the upper radial epiphysis, displacement of the entire distal humeral
epiphysis, and displacement of the capitellum which occur by direct
trauma and displacement of the olecranon epiphysis, the lateral epicondyle, and the medial epicondyle which may occur by avulsion forces.

These injuries are named for the epiphysis displaced and are further
amplified by application of our basic vocabulary related to epiphyseal
injuries.

Fractures of the Medial Epicondyle. Avulsion of the epiphysis of the medial epicondyle is common and is the result of a valgus strain applied to the elbow, with the force of the flexor group of muscles avulsing the epiphysis. In contrast, this same mechanism of injury in adults results in fractures of the radial head or neck.

The position of the avulsed fragment may range from minimal separation, to gross displacement with the epicondylar fragment being pulled into the joint between the humerus and the olecranon (Fig. II.154). Despite the amount of displacement, the injury is described as an avulsion fracture of the medial epicondyle.

Fractures of the Lateral Epicondyle. Displacement of the epiphysis of the lateral epicondyle usually includes the *capitellum*, resulting in a fracture which crosses the epiphyseal plate (Fig. II.155). This pattern is based on the mechanism of injury which usually results from a fall on the outstretched hand, so that the head of the radius is driven against the capitellum with the force continuing through the lateral condyle. Avulsion fractures also occur and are the result of severe varus

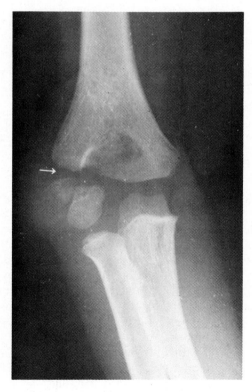

FIG. II.155. Fracture of the lateral epicondyle.

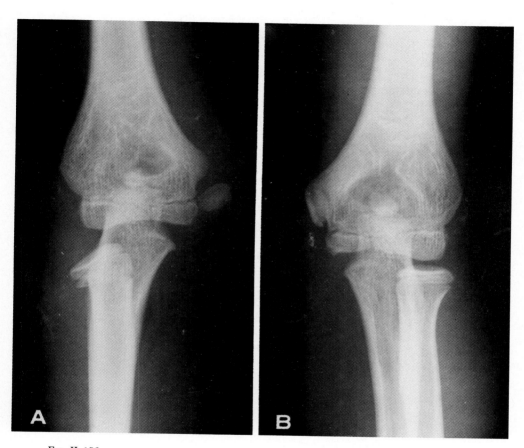

FIG. II.156.
(A) Separation of the proximal radial epiphysis with lateral displacement. The valgus force applied to the elbow also caused an avulsion of the medial epicondyle.
(B) Comparative view of the opposite elbow.

forces applied to the elbow. As previously stated, this injury may be readily identified on the anteroposterior projection but can present difficulty in interpretation on the lateral projection.

The capitellum is located anterior to the long axis of the humerus, forming an angle of approximately 45° with the shaft. Alteration in this angle occurs, when the lateral condyle is fractured and displaced, and, on the lateral projection, the displacement of the distal fragment is usually noted to be anterior.

The amount of displacement, however, is variable. The capitellum may be nondisplaced or rotated so that the fracture surface is directed outward and rotated in varying degrees up to as much as 180° by action of the forearm extensor muscles.

These injuries are described as lateral epicondylar fractures or fractures of the capitellum.

Intercondylar fractures and T fractures are comminuted fractures of the lower end of the humerus which are common in adults and very rare in children.

Fractures of the Proximal Ulna. In children, the strong pull of the triceps may result in a traction injury with avulsion of the olecranon epiphysis. The injury is simply described in the usual format for epiphyseal injuries.

Fractures of the Proximal Radial Epiphysis and Neck of the Radius. The valgus injuries to the elbow that produce fractures of the radial head and neck in adults and avulsion fractures of the medial epicondyle in young children also may displace the proximal radial epiphysis. This injury is described by the epiphysis involved and the amount and direction of angulation (Fig. II.156). Fractures of the radial neck in children are usually of the greenstick variety.

Dislocations of the Elbow

A variety of dislocations may occur at the elbow joint. These may involve the humeral articulation with the radius, the ulna, or both. Because of the intimate relation of the radius and ulna, a dislocation of one joint is usually accompanied by a fracture or dislocation of the adjacent bone.

Dislocation of the elbow *per se* usually refers to disruption of the humeroulnar articulation, with displacement of the proximal ulna, whereas disturbance of the humeroradial articulation is referred to as a dislocation of the radius.

Disruption of the Humeroulnar Articulation

In dislocations of the elbow, isolated displacement of the ulna is rare. More commonly, the radius maintains its normal relationship to the ulna and the two forearm bones are usually displaced backward, backward and outward, or backward and inward (Fig. II.157).

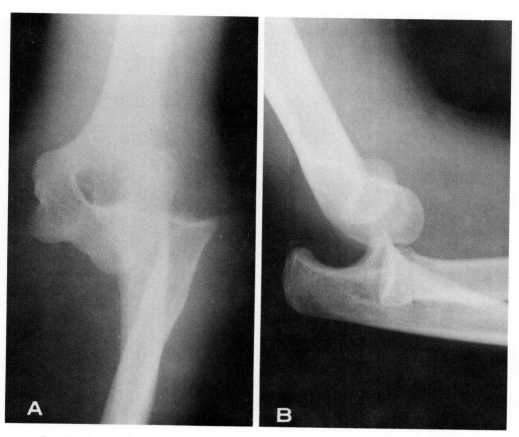

FIG. II.157 (A and B). Posterolateral dislocation of the elbow. Anteroposterior (A) and lateral (B) x-ray. The resting position of the ulna is posterior and lateral, thus the terminology of a posterolateral dislocation of the elbow. The radius has accompanied the ulna, maintaining their normal relationship.

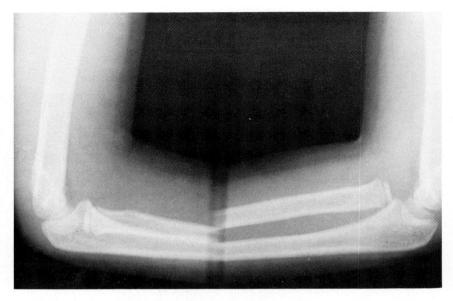

FIG. II.158. Anterior dislocation of the proximal radius on the right. Note that the ulna has maintained its normal anatomic position in relation to the trochlear. The comparative view shows the normal anatomy.

The dislocation is described by the residual position of the trochlear notch of the ulna in relation to the humerus. An anterior dislocation is one in which the trochlear notch is anterior to the humerus, whereas a posterior dislocation, which is much more common, is one in which the trochlear notch lies posterior to the condyles of the humerus. Lateral and medial dislocations also occur.

Dislocation of the Head of the Radius

Dislocation of the head of the radius occurs when there is a disruption of the humeroradial articulation. The description of the dislocation is by the relationship of the final resting position of the head of the radius to the humerus, as anterior, posterior, medial, or lateral (Fig. II.158). Divergent dislocations also occur, resulting when the head of the radius goes in one direction and the ulna in another.

Fracture Dislocations

Frequently dislocations of the elbow and radial head are associated with fractures. When a fracture complicates a dislocation, the pathology is described by the articulation dislocated, the residual position of the displaced bone, and by the anatomical location of the fracture. For example, a posterior dislocation of the elbow may be associated with a fracture of the coronoid process, a fracture of the head of the radius, or a fracture of the lateral condyle of the humerus, whereas a

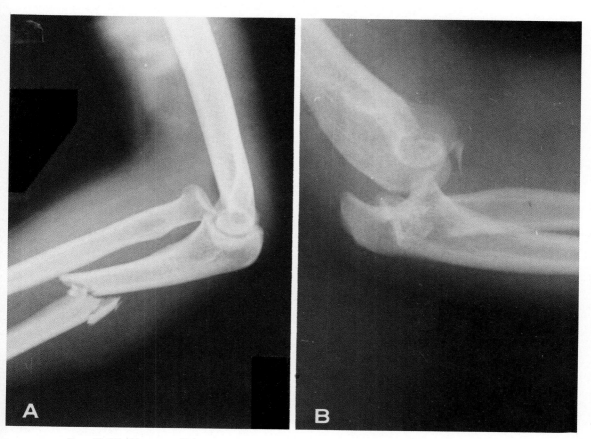

Fig. II.159. Fracture dislocation.

(A) Anterior dislocation of the head of the radius and a comminuted fracture of the junction of the proximal and middle thirds of the ulna.

(B) Posterior dislocation of the elbow with a transverse fracture of the neck of the radius and coronoid process. There also appears to be a linear fracture of the head of the radius.

dislocation of the head of the radius may be associated with fracture of the olecranon or a fracture of the shaft of the ulna (Fig. II.159).

Subluxation of the Head of the Radius

Subluxation of the head of the radius occurs in infancy and early childhood. The mechanism of injury is a traction force applied to the elbow, as when lifting a child by one hand when helping him from a curb. As a result of the trauma, the radial head is subluxated anteriorly, and the forearm is held in pronation. The diagnosis is based purely on clinical assessment as the radial head is unossified in the age group in which this injury occurs, and x-ray studies will not reveal the abnormality.

Review

Identify the fractures illustrated (Figs. A–G). Correct identification is given on page 386.

Figs. A–G.

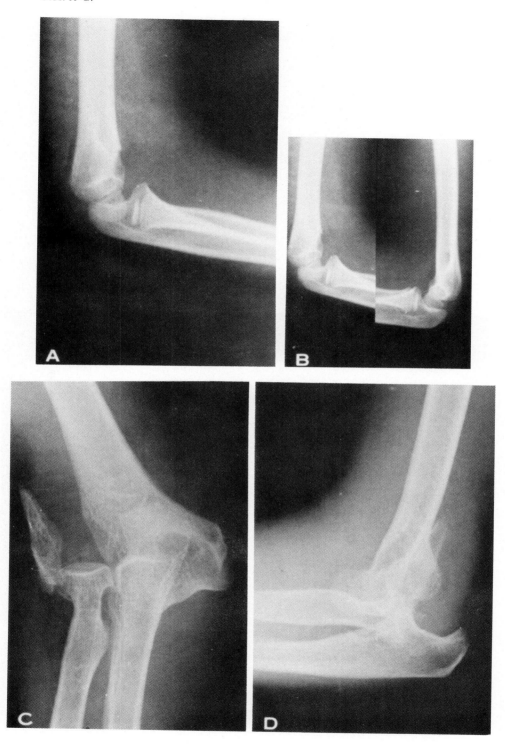

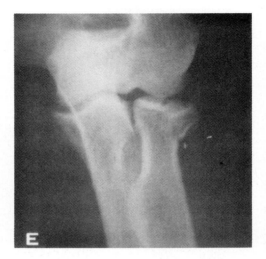

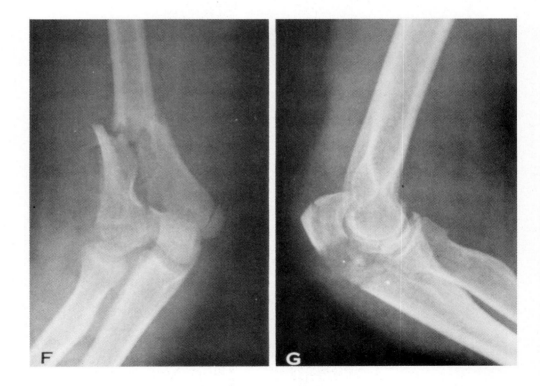

WRIST AND HAND

ANATOMY OF THE WRIST

The wrist is a synovial joint formed by the articulation of the distal radius, the carpal bones, and the metacarpals. The hub of the wrist or carpus is composed of eight short or cuboidal bones which are arranged roughly in two transversely oriented rows, a proximal and distal row of four bones each. The proximal row contains the carpal scaphoid (navicular), the lunate, triquetrum (triangular), and pisiform, and the distal row, the trapezium (greater multangular), the trapezoid (lesser multangular), the capitate, and the hamate. The proximal row of carpal bones articulates with the distal radius and the distal row articulates with the base of the metacarpals (Fig. II.160).

Thus three articulating rows may be designated: a radiocarpal joint, a midcarpal joint, and a carpometacarpal joint. The radiocarpal joint is the articulation between the radius and the proximal row of carpal bones, and the carpometacarpal joint, the articulation of the metacarpals with the distal row of carpal bones. The articulation between the proximal and distal row of carpal bones is called the midcarpal joint. The central portion of the midcarpal joint is formed by the articulation of the head of the capitate, with the cup-shaped concavity formed by the scaphoid and lunate.

The carpal bones are covered by cartilage on all articular surfaces which are mainly arthrodial or gliding in nature. The dorsal and palmar surfaces of the carpal bones are nonarticular, and serve for the attachments of the dorsal and palmar ligaments. These nonarticular areas of the bones have foramina for the entrance of blood vessels.

A fibrous capsule encloses the wrist joint and is reinforced by radial, ulnar, dorsal, and volar collateral ligaments. The synovial lining is extensive as it lines the joint capsule and extends between the adjacent carpal bones of each row.

There are no tendons inserted into any carpal bone. All the tendons cross the radiocarpal joint, the midcarpal joint, and the carpometa-

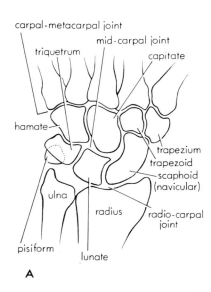

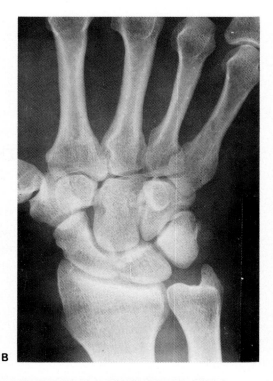

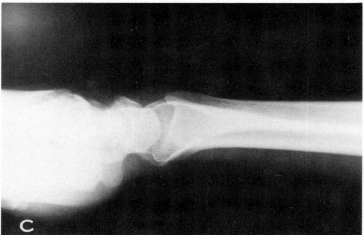

FIG.   II.160.
(A) Bony anatomy of the wrist. Note the radiocarpal, midcarpal, and carpometacar-pal joints.
(B and C) Anteroposterior (B) and lateral (C) radiographs of normal anatomy.

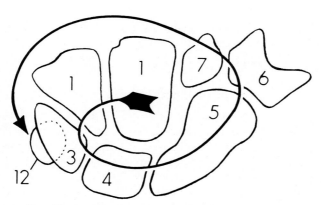

Fig. II.161. Schematic representation of the age of
onset, in years, of ossification of the carpus. (After
Grant.)

carpal joint, spanning the carpus to gain insertion into the metacarpals
and phalanges.

By means of these three transverse joints between the hand and the
forearm, plus the intercarpal joints, motion of the wrist occurs in every
direction to include flexion, extension, abduction (radial deviation),
adduction (ulnar deviation), and circumduction. The range of motion is
greater in adduction than abduction and flexion than extension. Predominantly, motion takes place at the radiocarpal and midcarpal joints,
with the carpometacarpal joint making only a minor contribution.
Abduction occurs mainly at the midcarpal joint (approximately 60–
65%) and adduction primarily at the radiocarpal joint (approximately
55–60%). Flexion occurs predominantly at the radiocarpal joint (65–
75%) and extension mainly at the midcarpal joint (75–85%). Circumduction occurs as a combination of the motions of abduction, adduction, flexion, and extension.

Ossification of the carpal bones takes place from a single center in
each bone, occurring quite consistently at a specific age. Consequently,
x-rays of the wrist to determine the extent of this ossification permits
one to determine the bone age of a child with reasonable accuracy. The
onset of ossification takes place in the following order: the capitate and
hamate ossify early in the 1st year of life, the capitate somewhat earlier
than the hamate. The triangular ossifies in the 3rd year. The lunate ossifies in the 4th or 5th year and the navicular in the 5th or 6th, followed
by the trapezium and the trapezoid during the 6th year of life.

The pisiform is a sesamoid bone which develops in the tendon of the
flexor carpi ulnaris and ossifies in the 12th year. Reflecting this dia-

grammatically reveals a somewhat spiral pattern which may assist in recalling the order of ossification (Fig. II.161).

INJURIES OF THE WRIST

Fracture of the Distal Radius and Ulna

Injuries to the distal radius and ulna are readily described by applying our basic vocabulary, noting the location, direction, comminution, and angulation or displacement of the fracture. The intraarticular nature of those fractures which extend into the wrist joint should also be noted. In two specific areas, fractures of the distal radius and ulna may be described by anatomic location. These are at the styloid processes, and fractures through these areas are designated as fractures of the radial or ulna styloid (Fig. II.162).

Injuries to Individual Carpal Bones

Carpal Navicular (Scaphoid)

Anatomy. The carpal navicular is named for its alleged resemblance to a boat. It is the largest bone of the proximal row of the carpus, and in most positions of the wrist, spans the midcarpal joint and tends to lie in both the proximal and distal row. The proximal surface of the carpal navicular is convex and articulates with the radius. The medial surface presents two articular facets, one for its articulation with the lunate, and the other, a large concavity, to accommodate part of the head of the capitate. A prominent tubercle is located in the distal palmar aspect of the bone and may be palpated at the base of the thumb. Arbitrarily, the carpal navicular may be divided into thirds which, for simplicity, may be designated as proximal, middle, and distal thirds; however, the more common nomenclature is that of proximal third, waist, and tubercle or distal pole (Fig. II.163).

Blood Supply. The arterial supply of the carpal navicular arises from branches of the radial and volar interosseous arteries. The vessels enter the navicular at two sites, through the lateral volar and dorsal surfaces near the waist, and at its distal aspect, the tubercle. Those that enter the tubercle supply primarily a circumscribed area in the distal part of the bone. The vessels that enter near the waist do so slightly distal to the center, and once through the cortical shell, divide and are directed predominately proximally and medially. These vessels supply the proximal two-thirds of the navicular. The proximal pole has no major vessels entering it but receives its blood supply from branches of the main arteries entering at the waist and also some vessels which are shared with the carpal lunate (Fig. II.164).

Fracture Nomenclature. Fractures of the navicular are of special interest to the orthopedic surgeon, stemming from the complications they present concerning union and avascular necrosis.

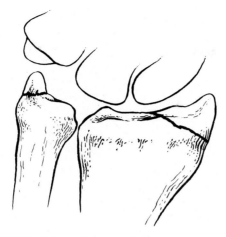

Fig. II.162. Oblique fracture of the styloid process of the radius and a transverse fracture of the styloid process of the ulna.

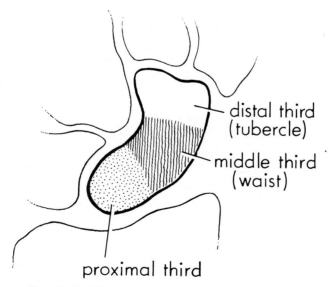

distal third (tubercle)

middle third (waist)

proximal third

Fig. II.163. For reference, the carpal navicular may be divided into thirds, namely proximal, middle, and distal.

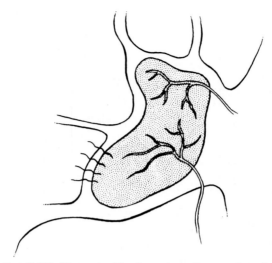

Fig. II.164. The major blood supply to the carpal navicular enters through the waist and distal pole. There are also some small vessels that are shared with the lunate.

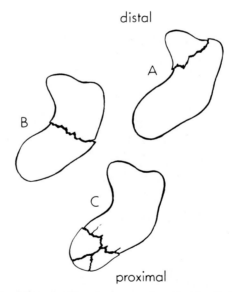

Fig. II.165. Fractures of the carpal navicular are described by their location; diagrammatically (A–C) and by radiographs (D–F).

    (A) Oblique fracture of the tubercle.
    (B) Transverse fracture of the waist.
    (C) Comminuted fracture of proximal pole.
    (D) Transverse fracture of the distal third.
    (E) Comminuted fracture of the waist.
    (F) Transverse fracture of the proximal pole.

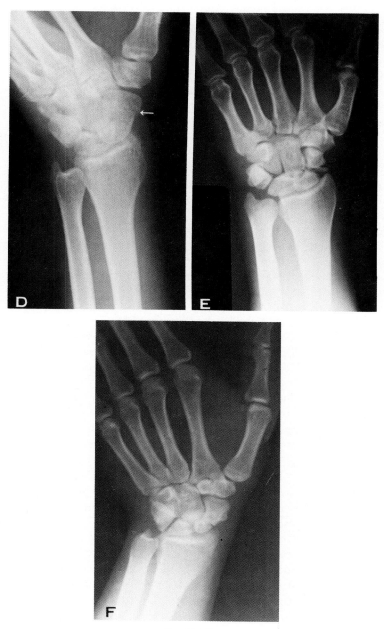

FIG. II.165

With the established reference points, there are essentially three anatomic levels where fractures of the navicular may occur: the tubercle, the waist, or the proximal pole. Fractures of the tubercle are located in the distal third of the bone, whereas fractures of the waist occur in the midportion of the bone. Fractures of the proximal pole occur in the proximal third of the navicular (Fig. II.165).

Fractures in any of these areas are described in routine fashion by their location, direction of the fracture, as transverse, oblique, comminuted, and amount of displacement of the fracture fragments.

It should be stressed that fractures of the navicular may be difficult to visualize on routine anteroposterior and lateral views of the wrist, and oblique views are essential. These fractures also may not be radiographically apparent immediately after the injury and only be visible following a period of 10–14 days, when bony reabsorption has taken place at the fracture site.

Complications of Fractures of the Carpal Navicular. The complications of fractures of the navicular encountered most frequently are those concerned with avascular necrosis of the proximal fragment and nonunion. As a general rule, the more proximal the fracture, the greater the incidence of complications.

Avascular necrosis. Avascular necrosis of the carpal navicular develops when the blood supply is interrupted by trauma. Initially, the bony architecture remains unchanged and the early roentgenographic pictures are normal. Later, the proximal fragment assumes an appearance of increased density when compared to the adjacent fragment (Fig. II.166). Studies should be continued over many months if the pathology is to be demonstrated. Fracture healing may take place despite the presence of avascular necrosis.

Nonunion of the carpal navicular. A certain number of carpal navicular fractures result in established nonunion. This may be the result of interruption of the arterial blood supply but, in addition, may be caused by missed or delayed diagnosis and treatment, which has resulted in inadequate immobilization. Nonunion may be recognized by a persistent radiolucent fracture line across the bone, sclerosis of the fracture margins, and, at times, cyst formation (Fig. II.167).

Fracture of the tubercle. Fractures of the tubercle are located in the distal third of the bone. Here both fragments have a free blood supply and union is certain, provided immobilization is adequate (Fig. II.168).

Fractures of the waist. Fractures of the waist occur near the midportion of the bone and, as a rule, both fragments have an independent blood supply. At times, depending upon whether the fracture is just distal or just proximal to the entrance of the vessels at the waist, the proximal fragment may suffer compromise of its blood supply. Fractures occurring distal to the entrance of the blood supply at the waist

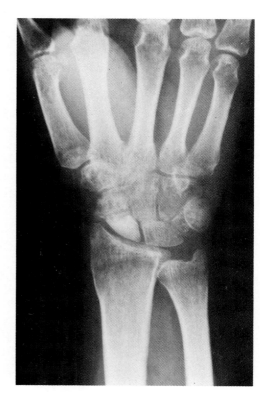

FIG. II.166. Avascular necrosis of the carpal navicular, following a transverse fracture through the waist. Note that the proximal fragment is relatively more dense than the surrounding bones. Nonunion of the fracture is also present.

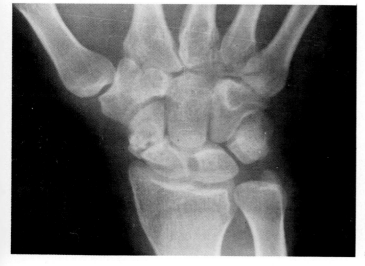

FIG. II.167. Nonunion following a transverse fracture through the waist of the carpal navicular. Note the persistence of the radiolucent fracture line, sclerosis of the fracture margins, and cyst formation. Despite the nonunion, both fragments have remained well vascularized and thus avascular necrosis has not occurred.

Fig. II.168. Fracture of the tubercle. These fractures pass between the entrance of the major vessels; thus both fragments are well vascularized.

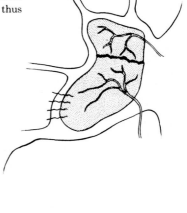

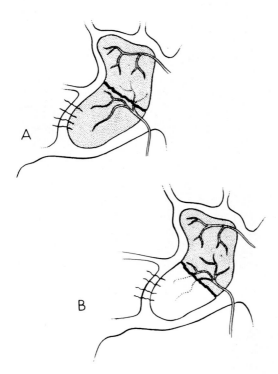

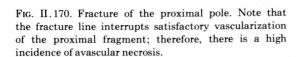

Fig. II. 169. Fractures of the waist present two possibilities.

(A) A fracture occurring distal to the entrance of the blood supply at the waist permits both fragments to be vascularized.

(B) Fracture occurring just proximal to the entrance of the blood supply at the waist interrupts the blood supply to the proximal fragment which then becomes poorly vascularized.

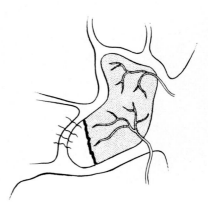

Fig. II.170. Fracture of the proximal pole. Note that the fracture line interrupts satisfactory vascularization of the proximal fragment; therefore, there is a high incidence of avascular necrosis.

do not interrupt the circulation to each fragment and thus permit both fragments to be vascularized (Fig. II.169A). Fractures occurring proximal to the entrance of the artery at the waist, however, interrupt the major blood supply to the proximal fragment which then becomes poorly vascularized (Fig. II.169B). When this occurs, nonunion and/or avascular necrosis may ensue. Thus fractures occurring through the proximal aspect of the waist carry with them an increased incidence of avascular necrosis of the proximal fragment and an increased incidence of nonunion as compared to fractures of the distal third.

Fractures of the proximal pole. Fractures of the proximal pole are fractures which occur in the proximal third of the navicular. These fractures carry a high incidence of avascular necrosis and nonunion because of compromise of the arterial blood supply to the proximal pole (Fig. II.170).

Thus, in addition to the basic nomenclature, these areas have marked clinical significance related to the blood supply to the bone.

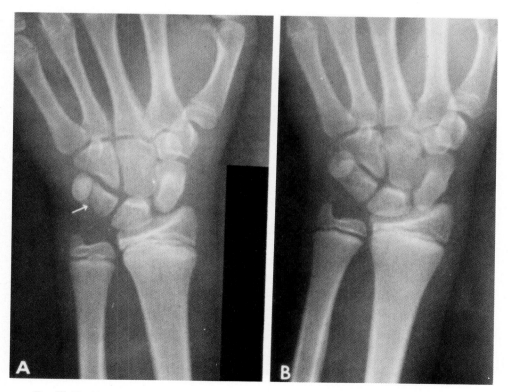

FIG. II.171 (A and B). Oblique fracture of the triquetrum. The opposite wrist is shown for comparison.

Fracture Nomenclature of Other Carpal Bones

Less common injuries are fractures to the other carpal bones which may be the result of direct trauma or avulsion forces. Description of these fractures is based on the individual carpal bone involved, using the basic nomenclature, for example, oblique fracture of the triquetrum (Fig. II.171).

Avulsion fractures of the carpus occur and are described as avulsion fractures of the particular bone involved. At times, because of the complexity of the architecture of the bones of the wrist noted on x-ray, the particular bone from which a fragment is avulsed is not easily or cannot be identified. Clinical examination may assist in the diagnosis (Fig. II.172).

Although the pisiform is a sesamoid bone, like the patella, fractures of the pisiform occur and are usually the result of a direct blow or fall in which the forces are directly applied to the hypothenar region. The fracture is usually a single transverse fracture, but at times may be comminuted. The injury is described as a fracture of the pisiform and amplified by other descriptive terminology.

DISLOCATIONS OF THE WRIST

A variety of dislocations may occur at the wrist. These may include disruption of the radiocarpal articulation with displacement of all the carpal bones or dislocations centered about individual carpal bones.

Displacement of the entire carpus is referred to as a dislocation of the wrist and is described by the final position of the carpal bones in relation to the radius. In a dorsal dislocation, the hand and carpus are displaced dorsally and proximally to rest on the dorsal surface of the radius. In a volar dislocation, the carpus is in contact with the volar surface of the radius (Fig. II.173).

Carpal Dislocations

Dislocations involving the bones of the two carpal rows usually occur from a fall on the extended wrist or outstretched hand. There are many varieties of dislocations and fracture dislocations of the carpus; however, this type of injury may be broken down into two major patterns:

1. Any carpal bone may be dislocated from the remaining carpus.
2. The rest of the carpus may be dislocated from a carpal bone which remains in its normal position.

Most commonly, dislocations of the wrist center about the lunate and the terminology applied to this bone may be applied to any of the carpal bones by substituting the name of the bone involved.

Lunate

Anatomy. The lunate lies just proximal to the most distal volar skin

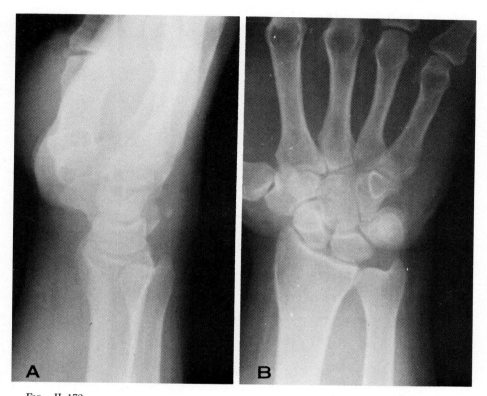

FIG. II.172.

(A) Avulsion fracture of the triquetrum. Note the difficulty in assessing from which bone the fracture arises.

(B) Anteroposterior x-ray offers little assistance.

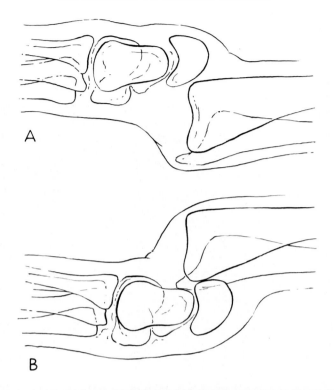

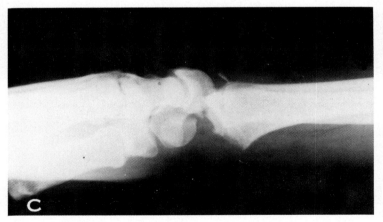

FIG. II.173. Dislocation of the wrist.

(A) Dorsal dislocation. The carpus is displaced dorsally in relation to the radius.

(B) Volar dislocation. The carpus is displaced volar to the radius.

(C) Radiograph of a dorsal dislocation associated with an avulsion fracture of the volar surface and a chip fracture of the dorsal surface of the distal radius.

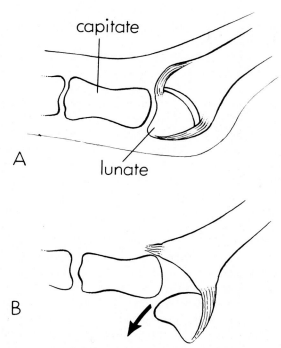

FIG. II.174 (A and B). Diagrammatic representation
of a dislocation of the lunate. Note that the lunate is
rotated on a capsular and ligamentous pedicle. (After
Watson-Jones).

crease of the wrist. It is semilunar or crescentic in shape with the concavity facing distally. Together with the concavity of the scaphoid, it forms a socket for the head of the capitate. The direction of its crescentic shape should be noted carefully for great importance lies in alteration that may occur with injury (Fig. II.160, page 260).

The two major types of injury previously mentioned occur in lunate dislocations, that is:

1. Dislocation of the lunate bone itself with the rest of the carpal bones remaining in their proper anatomic position (lunate dislocation).

2. Dislocation of the rest of the carpus where the lunate remains in its normal position (perilunate dislocation).

Dislocation of the Lunate. In this injury, the dislocated lunate is literally squeezed through the ligaments on the volar surface of the wrist and the remainder of the carpal bones remain in essentially normal alignment. The dislocated lunate may be rotated on a capsular and ligamentous pedicle anywhere from 90 to 270° (Fig. II.174).

Radiographically, the diagnosis of a dislocated lunate is made by noting a variation in the shape and position of the lunate. In the normal wrist, the concavity of the lunate faces distally when viewed from the side and, on anteroposterior projection, presents a somewhat quadrilateral appearance. When dislocated, the concavity of the lunate is found to be facing anteriorly or volarly on the lateral projection, whereas on the anteroposterior projection the lunate assumes a triangular shape in contrast to its normal somewhat quadrilateral shape (Fig. II.175). This injury is simply designated as dislocation of the lunate and the direction of the dislocation noted.

Perilunate Dislocation. In a perilunate dislocation, the lunate retains its normal relation to the distal end of the radius, while the other carpal bones are displaced, usually in a dorsal direction.

X-ray examination reveals disruption of the carpus. On anteroposterior projection, the lunate retains its somewhat quadrilateral shape and there is an overlapping shadow of the capitate and lunate not normally present. On the lateral view, the lunate is noted to retain its normal anatomic relationship to the radius with its concavity facing distally. The rest of the carpus is found to be displaced (Fig. II.176).

The injury is described as a perilunate dislocation, and the direction of displacement of the carpus should be specified.

Transcaphoid Perilunate Dislocation. Since the scaphoid bridges both the proximal and distal rows of carpal bones, it is susceptible to fracture, especially through the waist, when the rest of the carpus is being dislocated. Perilunate dislocations, therefore, are frequently associated with fractures through the waist of the scaphoid. In this injury,

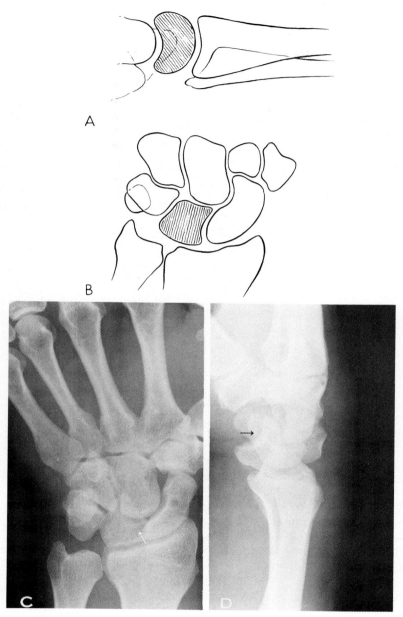

A

B

C

D

Fig. II.175. Dislocation of the lunate.

(A) In the normal wrist, the concavity of the lunate faces distally when viewed from the side.

(B) On anterorposterior projection, the normal lunate presents a somewhat quadrilateral shape.

(C) Radiograph of a lunate dislocation reveals, on anteroposterior projection, that the lunate assumes a triangular appearance in contrast to its usually quadrilateral shape.

(D) On lateral projection, the concavity of the lunate faces volarly and not distally.

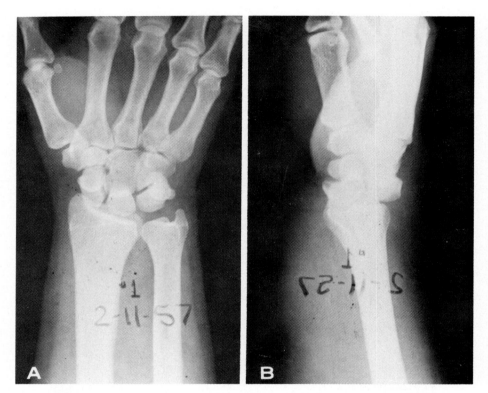

Fig. II.176.

(A) Perilunate dislocation with dorsal displacement of the carpus. Note that on the anterorposterior radiograph, the lunate retains its somewhat quadrilateral shape and there is overlap of the shadow of the capitate and the lunate.

(B) On the lateral view, the lunate has retained its normal relationship to the radius and the concavity is facing distally. The rest of the carpus is displaced dorsally.

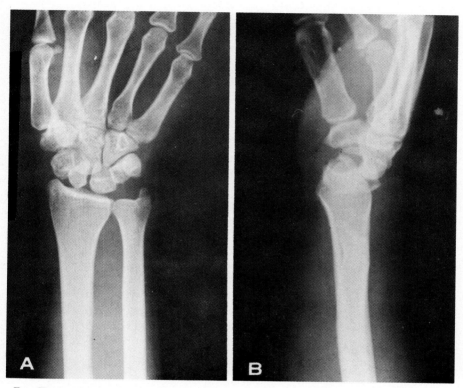

Fig. II.177 (A and B). Transcaphoid perilunate dislocation. Anteroposterior (A) and lateral (B) radiographs. The position of the lunate is similar to that of a perilunate dislocation. The scaphoid, however, is fractured and the proximal fragment has remained in its normal relationship to the lunate. The distal fragment is dislocated dorsally with the rest of the carpus. Note on the anteroposterior x-ray that the overlapping shadow of the capitate covers the lunate and the proximal navicular fragment.

the lunate and the proximal fragment of the carpal scaphoid remain in their normal relationship to the distal end of the radius, while the remainder of the carpus and distal fragment of the carpal scaphoid are displaced, most commonly, dorsally. The x-ray findings are similar to those found in a perilunate dislocation. On the anteroposterior view, the lunate retains its normal quadrilateral shape and position; however, it is now accompanied by the proximal fragment of the fractured navicular which also is in its normal position. The overlapping shadow of the capitate now covers the lunate and/or proximal fragment of the navicular. The lateral projection reveals the fracture of the navicular, and displacement of the rest of the carpus from the lunate accompanied by the distal fragment of the navicular (Fig. II.177).

This injury is designated as a transcaphoid perilunate dislocation.

Dislocations of the Other Carpal Bones

Dislocation of the other carpal bones occurs rarely; however, probably the most common of these rare dislocations is that of the scaphoid. When dislocated, the scaphoid is usually displaced volarly, and at times, quite distant from its normal anatomic position (Fig. II.178). A dislocation of any carpal bone is described in similar fashion to those of the lunate and scaphoid. Thus any fracture, dislocation, or combination of fracture and dislocation of the carpus may now be readily described. There may be dislocations or fractures of individual bones, or there may be dislocations of the rest of the carpus away from any of the individual carpal bones, such as periscaphoid lunate dislocation or transcapitate periscaphoid lunate dislocation. The terminology should include the name of the bone or bones involved, the direction of displacement, and a description of any accompanying fracture.

THE HAND

Fractures of Metacarpals and Phalanges

Metacarpals and phalanges are long bones, and fractures through these bones are described in the usual manner for long bones, as to location (proximal, middle, or distal thirds) and by the direction, type of angulation, as well as whether they are open or closed (Fig. II.179). At times, however, fractures of metacarpals and phalanges may be described by anatomic location. This occurs in two specific areas: (1) those in the proximal third may be described as fractures of the base of the metacarpal or phalanx and (2) fractures just proximal to the head can be described as fractures of the neck of the metacarpal or phalanx (Fig. II.180).

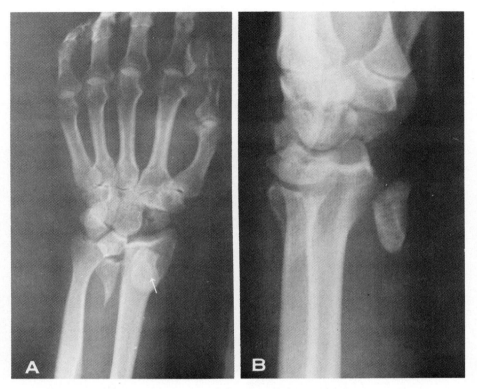

FIG. II.178 (A and B). Volar fracture dislocation of the scaphoid associated with fracture of the distal radius. Anteroposterior (A) and lateral views (B). Note that the scaphoid is widely displaced from its normal position. As with any dislocation of a carpal bone, the injury is named for the bone displaced and the direction of displacement.

Dislocations

Carpometacarpal joint, metacarpophalangeal joint, and interphalangeal joint dislocations may occur and are described by the joint involved and the final position of the distal bone in relation to the proximal one. These are usually dorsal or volar dislocations (Fig. II.181).

FRACTURES OF THE WRIST AND HAND IN CHILDREN

In general, fractures of the wrist and hand in children are described in similar fashion to adults; however, additional considerations must be made.

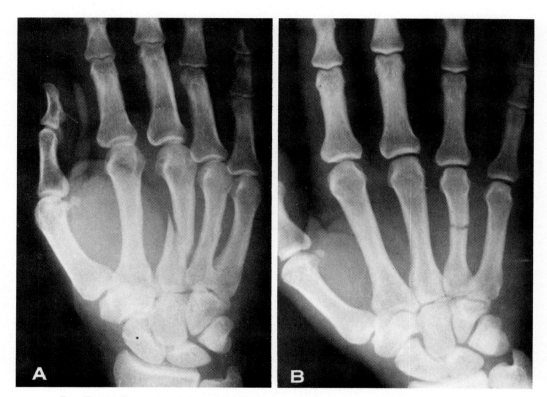

Fig. II.179. Fractures of the metacarpals are described in the usual manner for long bones.

(A) Oblique fracture of the junction of the proximal and middle third of the third metacarpal, and a nondisplaced oblique fracture of the middle third of the fourth metacarpal.

(B) Transverse fracture of the middle third of the fourth metacarpal.

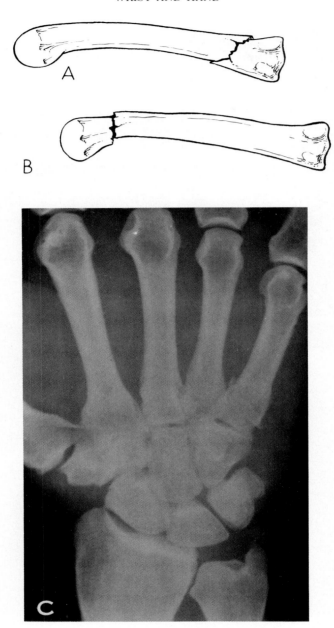

FIG. II.180.

(A) Diagrammatic representation of an oblique fracture through the base of the meta-carpal.

(B) Transverse fracture through the neck of the metacarpal.

(C) Radiograph of an oblique fracture of the base of the fifth metacarpal.

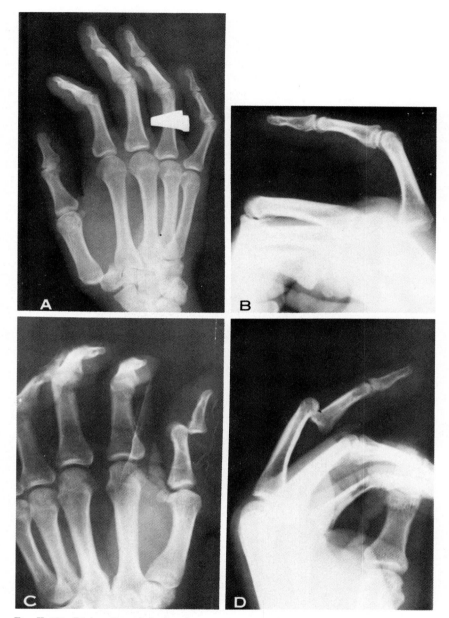

Fig. II.181. Dislocation of the hand.

(A) Carpal metacarpal dislocation. Radial dislocation of the first carpal metacarpal joint.

(B) Metacarpophalangeal joint dislocation. Dorsal dislocation of the metacarpophalangeal joint of the index finger.

(C) Dorsal dislocation of the interphalangeal joint of the thumb.

(D) Volar dislocation of the proximal interphalangeal joint of the middle finger. Note in each view, the direction of the dislocation is described by the resting position of the distal bone in relation to the proximal one.

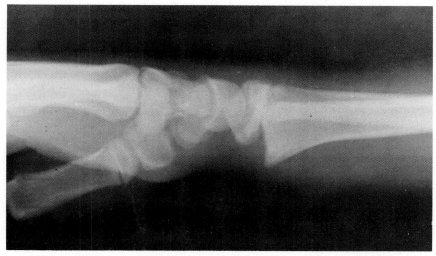

FIG. II.182. Separation of the distal radial epiphysis with a fracture of the metaphysis and dorsal displacement, or a Salter-Harris Type II epiphyseal injury of the distal radius.

Wrist

Prior to ossification, fractures and dislocations of carpal bones cannot be identified radiographically. Following ossification, comparative x-rays of the opposite extremity should be taken to assist in diagnosis.

In children, prior to epiphyseal closure, separation of the distal radial epiphysis occurs by the same mechanisms that produce fractures to the distal radius in adults. These injuries usually result in displacement of the entire radial epiphysis accompanied by a metaphyseal fragment and can be described in the usual manner for epiphyseal fractures (Fig. II.182).

Hand

A description of the epiphyses of the hand is interesting. The epiphyses of the phalanges of the thumb, index, middle, ring, and small fingers are located at the proximal aspect or base of the phalanx, while the epiphyses of the metacarpals of the fingers are located at the heads. A variation exists in the metacarpal of the thumb which presents a similar pattern to that of the phalanges with the epiphysis located at the base of the metacarpal (Fig. II.183). An awareness of the anatomic location of these epiphyses is essential to avoid mistaken diagnosis (see Section IV, page 350). Comparative x-rays will assist in proper evaluation.

Injuries to the epiphyses of the bones of the hand are described with routine vocabulary.

Review

Identify the fractures illustrated (Figs. A–H). Correct identification is given on page 387.

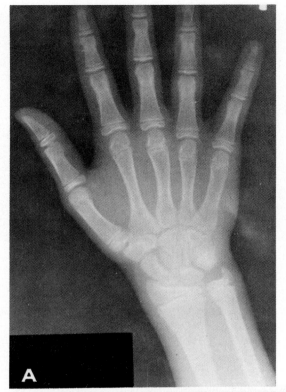

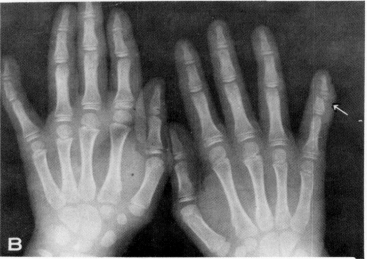

FIG. II.183.

    (A) Normal location of the epiphysis in a child's hand. Note the variation in the thumb metacarpal from the other metacarpals.

    (B) Transverse fracture of the distal third of the middle phalanx of the little finger. Note the similar appearance to an epiphyseal separation.

FIGS. A–D.

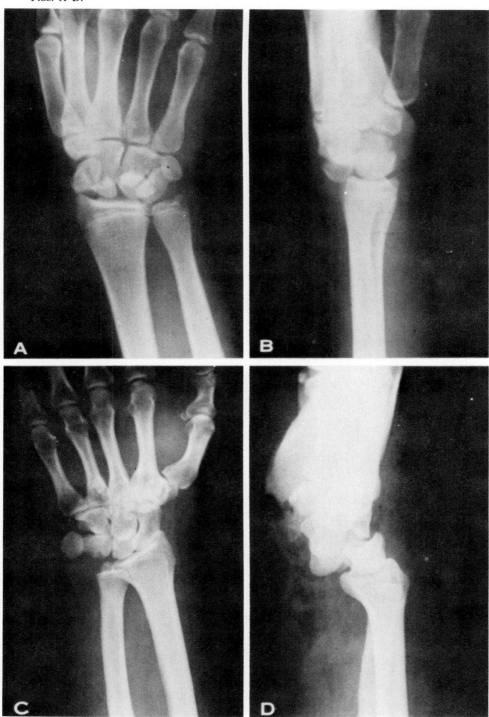

Figs. E–H.

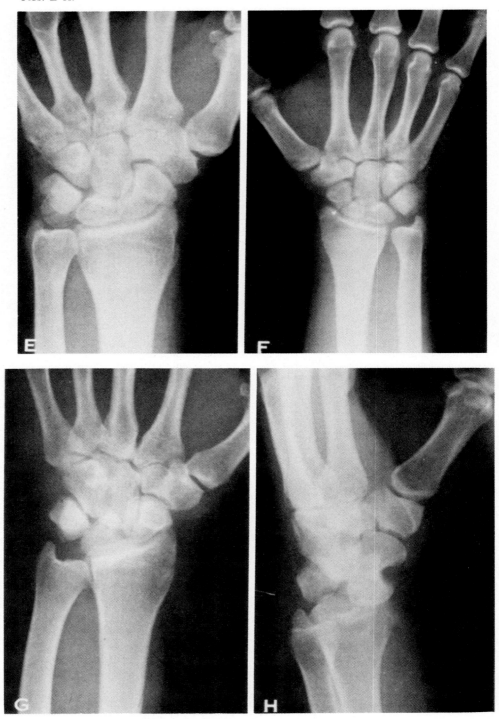

PART THREE

FRACTURE EPONYMS

Although, in recent years, eponymic description of disease processes has been discouraged and is laudably being discarded in favor of more precise anatomical, biochemical, or physiologic terminology, old habits die hard, and in orthopedics, in particular, an unusually large number of pathologic conditions continue to be identified by the more colorful and fanciful older method. While lending some charm, romance, and history to an otherwise precise and objective scientific discipline, unfortunately, these terms are frequently used inaccurately, and therein lies their greatest fault. Were they to mean the same thing to all people at all times, there would be little to gain by abandoning them, but through years of usage their meanings have frequently become nebulous, modified by additional pathology in some quarters, or strictly applied according to the original descriptions in others, so that terminologic precision in this area has suffered sadly.

Since it will take at least another generation, at best, to educate physicians in the use of the newer objective terms, it is anticipated that the use of the older eponymic descriptions will be with us for many years, and to the end that this latter terminology, if used, be used accurately and to mean the same thing to all physicians in all places and at all times, the following section is dedicated.

Many eponymic orthopedic terms were coined prior to the advent of the use of x-ray in 1885. The additional information gleaned from the use of this valuable diagnostic tool often revealed hitherto unsuspected associated pathology, consequently producing modification of the original description by one or more additional features.

In the following section, I shall define the eponymic term when possible based on the original description of the injury, and then, where necessary, supply further components which have been added through common usage or through the acquisition of subsequent information not available at the time of the original description.

Since both the recognition and appropriate use of eponymic terms promise to become more difficult, as this terminology falls into disuse, it is hoped that this section may provide a reliable reference source, enabling the reader to better comprehend and properly employ this colorful but dying nosology.

Aviator's Astragalus

"Aviator's astragalus" is a term that collectively refers to many varieties of fractures and fracture dislocations of the talus. The term was coined by Anderson in 1919, at which time he noted that fracture of the astragalus was comparatively rare in civilian life but quite common in aviation accidents. He felt that the trauma of aviation was usually the result of high velocity accidents, and fracture of the lower limbs, especially the talus, were relatively common.

The injury occurs as the aircraft strikes the ground at an angle so that the rudder bar, against which the instep of the foot is resting, is driven upward into the foot just in front of the heel. As a result, the astragalus absorbs most of the transmitted force and thus becomes the site of injury. Various mechanisms act upon the talus. The anterior edge of the distal tibia can act as a fracturing agent, or torsional forces can be applied to the talus due to the momentum carrying the pilot forward. In addition, one side of the foot may receive more force than the other, depending on the angle that the plane strikes the ground. The position of the foot prior to fracture is also variable, being either in a position of acute dorsiflexion, plantar flexion, or inversion. This variety of foot positions and forces produces a variety of fractures of the astragalus, that include compression fractures of the neck, fractures of the body or posterior processes, or fractures associated with dislocations, all of which are considered in the group designated as "aviator's astragalus."

Barton's Fracture

Barton's fracture is a fracture of the dorsal articular margin of the distal radius with the separated fragment, containing a margin of articular cartilage, being displaced upward and backward onto the dorsal surface of the radius (Fig. III.1).

This fracture occurs from a fall on the outstretched hand with the hand being violently bent backward, driving the carpus against the dorsal margin of the articular surface of the radius. The resulting displacement of the detached fragment may range from minimal to signif-

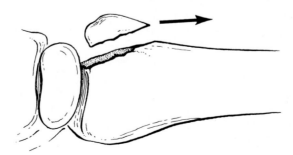

Fig. III.1. Barton's fracture.

icant, and if sufficient displacement does occur, the carpus follows the radial fragment with a resultant dorsal subluxation (Fig. III. 2).

This fracture was described by John Rhea Barton in 1838 to distinguish an intermediate injury between a sprain and a dislocation of the wrist. He believed that although the lesion had characteristics of both sprains and dislocations, it was distinguishable from either. He also separated this injury from fractures of the radius, or radius and ulna, occurring proximal to the joint without joint involvement. He described the pathology and clinical findings prior to the advent of x-ray, based solely on clinical observations.

At times, fractures of the volar articular margin of the distal radius are referred to as reverse Barton's fractures (Fig. III. 3). This term should probably be changed to a Barton's fracture involving the volar or anterior articular margin as Barton gave an anatomic description of this lesion in his original article. He noted that, although rare, a fracture may occur on the palmar side of the radius secondary to a force applied against the back of the hand. This injury, he stated, usually occurs "in awkward attempts to parry the blow from a fist, from pressure in dense crowds and from falling on the back of the hand whilst it is bent forward."

Baseball Finger (Mallet Finger)

A baseball or mallet finger is a flexion deformity of the distal phalanx. The lesion is produced by a blow, commonly caused by being struck on the fingertip by a baseball, resulting in forced flexion of the distal phalanx and separation of the common extensor tendon from its insertion into the base of the distal phalanx. This tendon separation occurs either through rupture of the tendon itself or avulsion of a fragment of bone from the dorsum of the base of the distal phalanx into which the tendon inserts. The result is a flexion deformity of the distal phalanx of approximately 30° with inability to actively extend the tip of the finger (Fig. III. 4).

Bennett's Fracture

Bennett's fracture is a fracture of the base of the first metacarpal, involving the proximal articular surface. It presents as an oblique fracture involving the carpometacarpal joint in such a way that a triangular fragment of bone from the first metacarpal is separated from the remaining portion of the metacarpal and remains in its normal position, articulating with the greater multangular. The major fragment or shaft of the metacarpal is displaced proximally, with its dorsal surface intact (Fig. III. 5). The result is thus a fracture through the base of the metacarpal with proximal dislocation of the metacarpal shaft.

This fracture was described by Edward Hallinan Bennett in 1881, when, prior to the advent of x-ray, he described fractures of the meta-

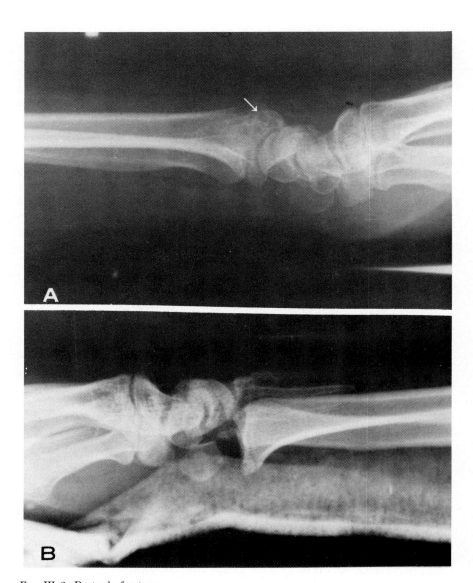

FIG. III.2. Barton's fracture.
   (A) Without displacement.
   (B) Similar fracture with displacement of the dorsal fragment and subluxation of the carpus.

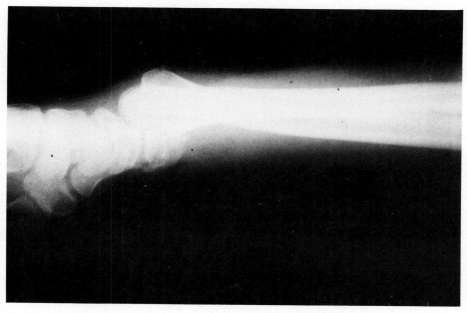

FIG. III.3. Barton's fracture involving the volar articular margin.

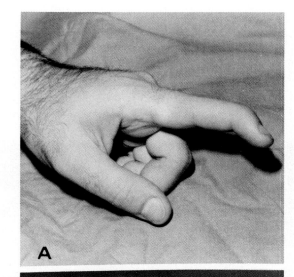

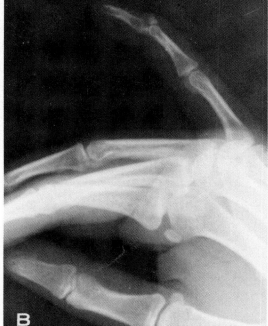

FIG. III. 4. Baseball finger (mallet finger).
   (A) Clinical deformity of the mallet finger.
   (B) Radiograph of an avulsion fracture from the dorsum of the base of the distal phalanx. The soft tissue
outline demonstrates the flexion deformity of the distal
phalanx.

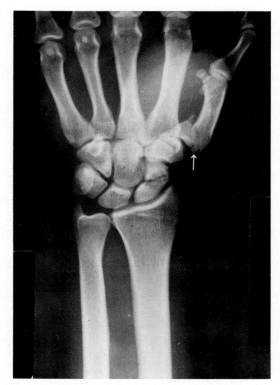

Fig. III.5. Bennett's fracture. Note that the triangular fragment has remained in its normal position and the shaft is displaced proximally with its dorsal surface intact. A fracture of the carpal navicular is also present.

carpal bones based on anatomic dissections of specimens and clinical observations in patients. He presented a series of united fractures of the metacarpals with the object of determining the character and site of the most frequent fractures of these bones. He noted that the first and fifth metacarpal were most frequently involved, but felt that what was of greater interest was the site and character of involvement of the first metacarpal. In his series, the metacarpals of the thumb had changes on the proximal articular surface, which represented the oblique fracture which passed through the base of the bone, detaching the largest part of the articular surface from the small piece supporting it.

He clinically confirmed his findings by noting the outward appearance of a subluxated thumb, and further stressed the importance of measurements of the dorsal surface of the metacarpal in evaluating the extent of the fracture. Since no measurable shortening of that surface was present, it indicated that the dorsal surface was not fractured.

Boxer's Fracture

A boxer's fracture is a fracture of the neck of the fifth metacarpal. The fracture occurs as a result of a direct blow against the fifth metacarpal head with the fist clenched, in similar fashion that a fighter uses to deliver a blow. The result is dorsal angulation at the fracture site with the head of the metacarpal being displaced volarly into the palm (Fig. III.6).

Bumper Fracture (Fender Fracture of the Tibia at the Knee)

A bumper or fender fracture, described by Cotton in 1929, is a compression fracture of the lateral tibial plateau, resulting in separation of the margin of the plateau or depression of the central portion of the articular surface (Fig. III.7).

The fracture is produced by forced abduction of the leg at the knee, when the tire, bumper, or fender of a vehicle strikes its lateral aspect with the leg in extension and the foot fixed on the ground. The result is that the lateral femoral condyle and the tibial plateau are forcibly driven together by the valgus stress. The femoral condyle, being much harder, causes the softer tibial plateau to give way, producing a comminuted depressed fracture of the lateral tibial plateau.

Chance Fracture

A Chance fracture is a vertebral fracture in which there is a horizontal splitting of the spinous process and neural arch, ending with an anterior extension directed in an upward curve which usually reaches the upper surface of the body just in front of the neural foramen (Fig. III.7.1).

The lesion was described by G. Q. Chance in 1948 as a rare fracture caused by a flexion injury to the spine. Most commonly, an acute flexion injury to the spine results in a compression fracture of the vertebral body. If, however, for some reason the body is relatively incompressable, there now occurs disruption of the posterior elements and the above fracture can result.

Although slight wedging of the vertebral bodies may result, there is no tendency to dislocation nor cord damage.

Chauffeur's Fracture (Backfire Fracture, Lorry Driver's Fracture)

A chauffeur's fracture or backfire fracture is an oblique fracture of the distal radius in which the fracture line extends radially from the articular surface, separating a triangular portion of bone including the styloid process from the main bone (Fig. III.8).

The fracture occurs when, while cranking a car, a backfire occurs and

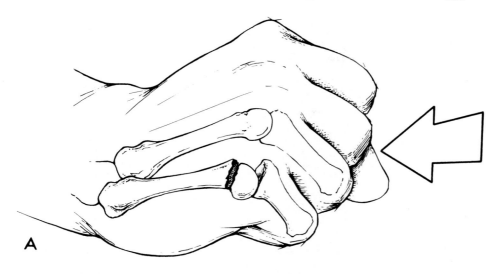

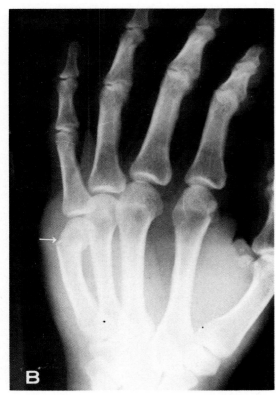

FIG. III.6. Boxer's fracture.
(A) Mechanism of injury.
(B) Radiograph.

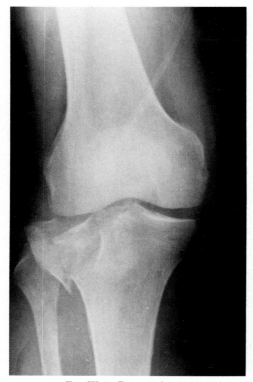

FIG. III.7. Bumper fracture.

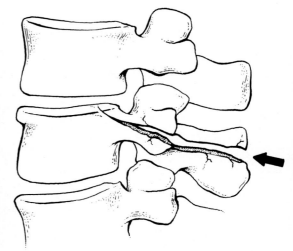

FIG. III.7.1. Chance fracture (after Chance).

places a terrific force on the starting handle. Two mechanisms then produce the injury, one direct and the other indirect, and result in several types of fractures, each probably with the right to be called a chauffeur's fracture. The direct trauma is produced when the crank flies out of the hand, strikes the forearm, and causes a fracture at the site of impact. The indirect method occurs without the handle leaving the hand. When the handle kicks back sharply, it forces the hand and wrist into dorsiflexion and abduction producing the triangular fragment involving the styloid process of the distal radius which carries the name chauffeur's fracture.

Chisel Fracture

A chisel fracture is an incomplete fracture of the head of the radius in which the fracture line extends distally from the center of the articular surface, approximately ½ inch (Fig. III.9).

Chopart's Fracture and Dislocation

Chopart's dislocation or fracture dislocation is an injury involving the midtarsal joints (talonavicular and calcaneal cuboid joints) of the foot (Fig. III.10). Although the fracture was not described by Chopart, the

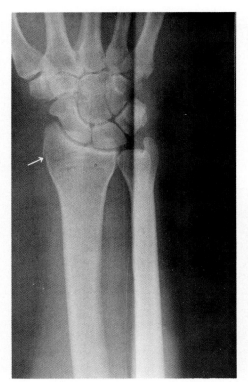

Fig. III.8. Chauffeur's fracture. Note the fracture of the distal radius extending radially from the articular margin, separating the styloid process.

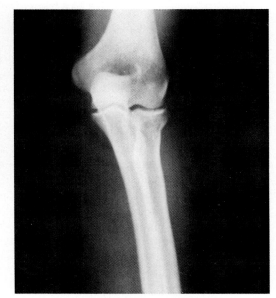

Fig. III.9. Chisel fracture.

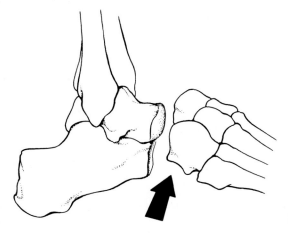

Fig. III.10. Chopart's fracture.

midtarsal joints have been referred to as Chopart's joints as a result of his description of a method of amputation of the foot through the midtarsal region, and subsequently the fracture term was applied.

The injury is usually the result of severe direct trauma in the form of crushing or compression injury. Commonly there is medial displacement of the distal fragments at the midtarsal joint with the foot displaced inward and upward, although displacement can occur in other directions. Dislocation, as an isolated injury, is rare and almost never occurs, but is usually associated with bony avulsions from the cuboid, navicular, and calcaneus.

Clay-Shoveler's Fracture

A clay-shoveler's fracture is a fracture of one or more spinous processes of the lower cervical or upper thoracic vertebrae (Fig. III.11).

In 1933, large numbers of previously unemployed men were given jobs digging drainage troughs through clay soil in swampy areas in southwestern Australia. A great proportion of these workers were not used to heavy work, or perhaps any work at all. In digging the drains the clay had to be tossed up 10, 12, or 15 feet with long-handled shovels. The injury occurred when the worker attempted to throw up a shovel full of clay and the clay stuck to the shovel. This sudden and unexpected check exerts a force opposite to the neck muscles. As a result of either direct muscle or reflex muscle contracture, or pull through the supraspinous ligament, the worker experienced an acute onset of pain, and, at times, an audible crack followed by the inability to continue working.

The fracture most commonly occurs at the spinous process of the seventh cervical vertebra; however, the sixth cervical to the third thoracic vertebrae may be involved. At times, two adjacent vertebrae may be involved.

Colles' Fracture

Fractures of the distal radius comprise the majority of fractures of the wrist and, in the light of Colles' original description, many are loosely referred to as Colles' fractures. Recently this term has come to describe fractures of the distal radius within 1 inch of the articular margin, with dorsal displacement of the distal fragment and volar angulation accompanied by shortening (Fig. III.12). In some instances, the description has even been extended to include fractures which extend into the radiocarpal joint.

Much of our modification of the features of the Colles' fracture has come about because of roentgenographic studies. The status of the distal ulna, for example, is always mentioned in Colles' fractures because, in association with fractures of the distal radius, the styloid process may be pulled off, the triangular fibrocartilage ruptured, or the

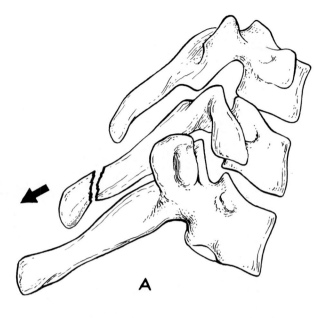

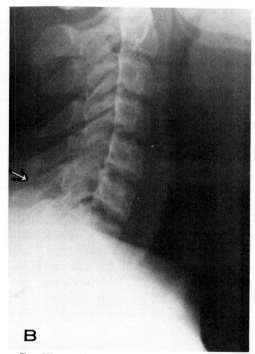

FIG. III. 11. (A and B) Clay-shoveler's fracture.

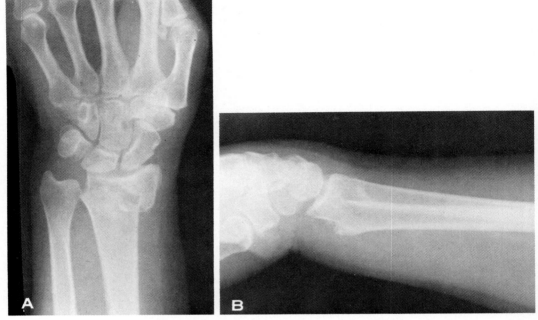

Fig. III.12. (A and B) Colles' fracture—antero-posterior (A) and lateral (B) x-ray.

head of the ulna displaced. The original description by Abraham
Colles, which was before the advent of x-ray, however, described the
status of the ulna only as being prominent, "projecting toward the
palm and inner edge of the limb; the degree, however, in which this
projection takes is different in different instances."

Abraham Colles in 1814 described the fracture (which he considered
the most common injury of the wrist) as a fracture of the distal radius
which occurred about 1½ inches proximal to the joint, with dorsal and
upward displacement of the distal articular surface, with palmar and
medial prominence of the distal ulna and rupture of the supporting ligaments of the distal radioulnar articulation. His purpose was to differentiate this lesion based on clinical experiences from a sprain or a dorsal
dislocation of the carpus which it so closely resembled. Without x-ray,
the difficulty in making the diagnosis was due to the absence of crepitus (because of impaction) which was a common finding in fractures;
the constant recurrence of the deformity following reduction which was
inconsistent with the diagnosis of dislocation; and the persistence of
deformity after the swelling had subsided which did not occur in
sprains.

Presently, Colles' fracture is a loose term applied to fractures of the
distal radius, with or without an accompanying ulna styloid fracture, in

which there is dorsal displacement of the distal fragment.

Fractures of the distal radius with volar displacement of the distal fragment, although not described by Colles, have been called reverse Colles' fractures (see "Smith's Fracture," page 323).

Cotton's Fracture

Cotton's fracture is a trimalleolar fracture of the ankle which includes fractures of both malleoli and the posterior articular margin of the distal tibia (posterior malleolus) with the latter fragment being displaced posteriorly and/or superiorly (Fig. III.13).

The fracture was described by Frederick Cotton in 1910 as a tibial fracture in which the fracture line separates the medial malleolus and continues backward, separating the entire posterior distal tibial articulating surface, and, in addition, has an associated fracture of the fibula just above the ankle joint. As the attachments of the posterior capsule to the talus and distal tibia are not ruptured, posterior subluxation of the talus accompanies displacement of the medial malleolus and the posterior malleolar fragment, all of which are drawn up behind the tibia.

Cotton initially referred to the lesion as a Pott's fracture associated with a fracture of the posterior articular surface of the tibia, inasmuch as he felt the term Pott's fracture was generally used for many ankle injuries which he realized were different than what Pott originally described. He stressed, however, that this fracture had a great tendency toward recurrence, and thus considered the lesion to be very serious. This feature specifically caused him to consider this fracture, although classified as a variant of Pott's fracture, to be a separate entity.

Dashboard Fracture

A dashboard fracture is a fracture of the posterior rim of the acetabulum. The name is derived from the mechanism of injury, whereby the seated automobile passenger, at the moment of impact, is thrown forward, striking the dashboard with his knee and transmitting the force up the femur, so that the head of the femur is driven against the posterior rim of the acetabulum (Fig. III.14).

deQuervain's Fracture

deQuervain's fracture is a fracture dislocation of the wrist in which the carpal scaphoid is fractured and the proximal fragment, accompanied by the lunate, is dislocated volarward (Fig. III.15).

The lesion was described in 1907 by F. deQuervain when he noted that, in addition to the fullness usually produced by a palmar dislocation of the lunate, there was tenderness over the scaphoid, shortening of the carpus, and radial displacement of the hand. He termed this injury a "typical intercarpal dislocation fracture."

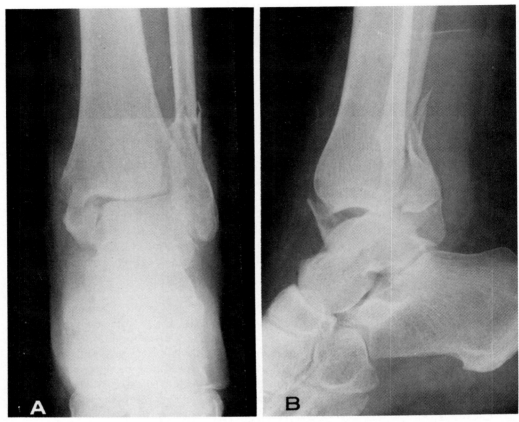

FIG. III.13. (A and B) Cotton's fracture or trimalleolar fracture—anteriorposterior (A) and
lateral (B) x-ray.

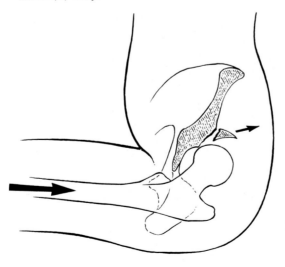

FIG. III.14. Dashboard fracture.

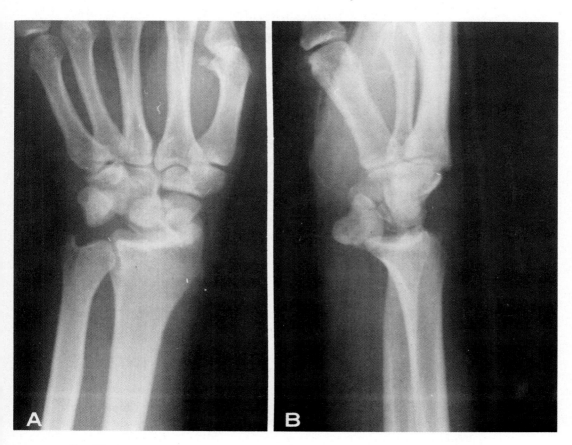

FIG. III.15. (A and B) deQuervain's fracture—anteroposterior (A) and lateral (B) x-ray. Note on the anteroposterior radiograph the transcaphoid fracture, with the distal fragment remaining in its proper anatomic position and the proximal fragment of the scaphoid and lunate poorly outlined. On the lateral view, volar displacement of the lunate and proximal fragment of the scaphoid is apparent and the remainder of the carpus is in its normal anatomic position.

A deQuervain's fracture should not be confused with the more common transcaphoid perilunate dislocation in which the lunate and the proximal fragment of the navicular retain their normal position, and the rest of the carpus, accompanied by the distal fragment of the scaphoid, is displaced backward.

Desault's Dislocation of the Wrist

Desault's dislocation describes primarily a volar displacement of a dislocation of the distal radius.

The lesion was described by P. J. Desault prior to 1805, at which time, based on patient evaluation and the reproduction of the traumatic forces of supination and pronation on cadaver specimens, he described the mechanism of injury and clinical findings of "subluxation" of the distal radius. He noted that volar "subluxation" was produced by forced pronation of the radius, resulting in a dorsal prominence produced by the head of the ulna and a volar mass produced by anterior displacement of the distal end of the radius. On the other hand, "subluxation" of the radius dorsally, was produced by forced supination and characterized by a volar mass produced by the ulna associated with dorsal displacement of the distal end of the radius. He further described other characteristics of the deformities, but emphasized that these injuries must not be mistaken for sprains.

He felt that volar subluxation of the distal radius occurred frequently and that dorsal displacement was rare, stating he had seen it only once.

Although not commonly used at the present time, the eponym is one to which Colles referred for comparison in stressing the frequency of fractures of the distal end of the radius.

Dupuytren's Fracture

Dupuytren's fracture, as classically described, is a fracture of the distal fibula (lateral malleolus), with rupture of the distal tibiofibular ligaments, diastasis of the syndesmosis, lateral dislocation of the talus, and displacement of the foot upward and outward (Fig. III. 16).

Presently, Dupuytren's fracture is used to describe several varieties of bimalleolar fractures, but most commonly those caused by abduction and external rotation forces that result in an avulsion fracture of the medial malleolus and an oblique fracture of the lateral malleolus with or without rupture of the tibiofibular syndesmosis. This varied use of the term, Dupuytren's fracture, is the result of his wide descriptions of many fractures of the ankle. In some instances, the eponym has been used synonymously with Pott's fracture.

The fracture was described as a rare lesion by Dupuytren, based on a

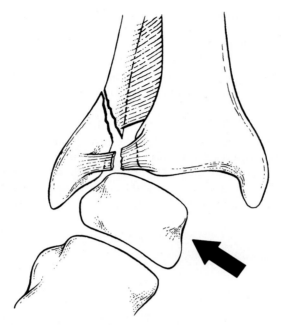

FIG. III.16. Dupuytren's fracture.

single clinical case in 1816 in which a patient who had sustained a fracture of the distal fibula also presented with a widened ankle mortice and medial displacement of the tibia, with the talus, foot, and lateral malleolus displaced laterally two thumb lengths above their normal position. To produce these clinical findings, he concluded that the fractured fibula was accompanied by rupture of the ligaments connecting the tibia and the fibula and that the force of the foot dislocating outward and upward displaced the lateral malleolus.

As originally described, the lesion appears similar to the ankle injury described by Pott, except that Dupuytren mentions rupture of the tibiofibular syndesmosis and Pott the medial ligaments of the ankle. This may also account for their interchangeable use at the present time (see "Pott's Fracture," page 318).

Essex-Lopresti's Fracture

An Essex-Lopresti's fracture is a comminuted fracture of the head of the radius, associated with dislocation of the distal radioulnar joint.

The injury was described in 1951 by Peter Essex-Lopresti as a rare condition produced by a violent longitudinal compression force in the long axis of the radius, this mechanism of injury being different than the more common injury of forced abduction at the elbow which usually produces fractures of the radial head.

Galeazzi's Fracture

Galeazzi's fracture is a fracture of the radius at the junction of the middle and distal thirds, associated with subluxation of the distal ulna (Fig. III. 17).

The fracture was described by Ricardo Galeazzi in 1935, at which time he noted the similarity of this fracture to the Monteggia fracture, in mechanism of injury and pathology, with one bone remaining intact and the other being fractured. He felt that the shortening of the radius predisposed the distal ulna or radioulnar joint to subluxation or dislocation, at times being associated with fracture of the ulna styloid.

Gosselin's Fracture

Gosselin's fracture is a V-shaped fracture of the distal tibia.

The lesion was described by Leon Gosselin in 1855 in an attempt to clinically differentiate the entity from the more common oblique fracture of the tibia. Based on clinical examination and autopsy dissection, he described the fracture as a V-shaped lesion in which the apex of the "V" faces distally, so that the proximal fragment is pointed and is received in the V-shaped groove of the distal fragment. An associated fissure fracture may be present, extending distally from the tip of the "V" of the distal fragment to the medial aspect of the shaft of the tibia, and then continuing posteriorly, ending at the distal tibial articular surface (Fig. III. 18).

He felt that the fracture was very unstable, and since the point of the proximal fragment was very sharp, a compound wound could easily occur.

Greenstick Fracture

A greenstick fracture is an incomplete angulated fracture producing a bowing of the bone. It derives its name from that of breaking a young branch which snaps on its outer surface but is maintained intact on its inner surface (see "Greenstick Fracture," page 52).

Hangman's Fracture of the Cervical Spine

A hangman's fracture is a traumatic lesion characterized by a bilateral avulsion fracture through the lamina or pedicles (neural arch) of the second cervical vertebra (axis), without injury to the odontoid process and with or without dislocation of the body of the axis on the third cervical vertebra (Fig. III. 19). Although these fractures are com-

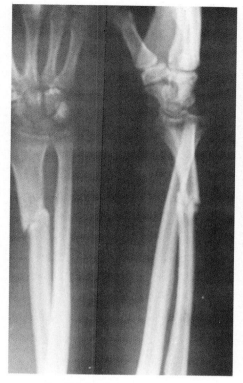

FIG. III. 17. Galeazzi's fracture.

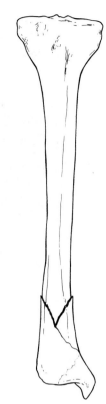

FIG. III. 18. Gosselin's fracture.

monly the result of high-velocity trauma, the descriptive terminology
derives from the similar pathology produced by the current mode of
hanging that employs the use of the submental knot.

Hanging was first introduced into 5th century England, but without
standardization of techniques, death ensued primarily from strangula-
tion. Later refinements led to the development of the long drop and
eventually the use of the submental knot which invariably leads to
avulsion fracture through the neural arch of the axis.

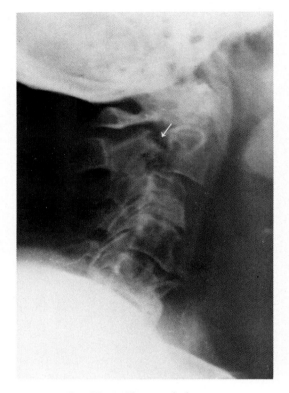

FIG. III.19. Hangman's fracture.

Jefferson's Fracture

Jefferson's fracture is a comminuted fracture of the ring of the atlas, sometimes referred to as a bursting fracture of C-1. The fracture, as described in 1919 by Godfrey Jefferson, is produced by a severe compressive force directed downward to the top of the head resulting in transmitted force from the head via the occipital condyles to the cervical spine, so that the atlas is compressed between the skull and the axis. The net result of the crush produces divergent forces from the occiput and C-2, causing separation and lateral spread of the two lateral masses, and a fracture in one or more segments of the atlas ring (Fig. III.20).

Kocher's Fracture

Kocher's fracture is an osteochondral fracture of the capitellum which results in a separation of a semilunar fragment of the articular

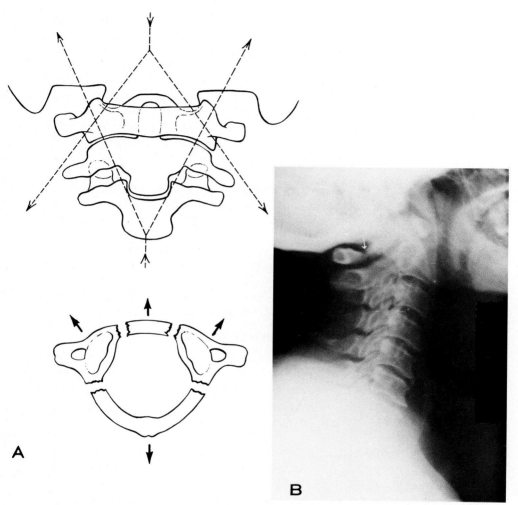

Fig. III.20. Jefferson's fracture (after G. Jefferson, *British Journal of Surgery*, 7: 416, 1920).

(A) Net result of the crush produces divergent forces upon the atlas and a bursting of the ring.

(B) Radiograph.

cartilage and the underlying bone. The dislodged fragment is usually displaced into the joint.

Le Fort's Fracture

Le Fort's fracture is a vertical fracture of the anterior medial margin of the distal fibula (Fig. III.21).

The lesion was described by Leon Le Fort in 1886, as a vertical avulsion fracture involving the medial aspect of the lateral malleolus, at the insertion of the inferior tibiofibular ligament. He presented a study of four patients whom he felt did not have the characteristic findings present in the ordinary avulsion fractures of the lateral malleolus. When these patients were first seen, he thought he was treating a sprain of the ankle; however, the slow response to treatment caused him to investigate further and more critically localize his physical findings.

The mechanism of injury was described as an adduction injury to the ankle which placed a great amount of tension on the inferior tibiofibular ligament, causing the fragment of bone to be avulsed by the tibiofibular ligament, if the ligament itself did not rupture.

Describing the vertical direction of the fracture without radiographs was empirically based on the relatively rapid recovery, the stable mortice, and the lack of abnormal findings present on extension or flexion of the ankle, all of which he felt were not the findings usually associated with transverse fractures of the fibula.

Lisfranc's Fracture Dislocation

Lisfranc's joint is the tarsometatarsal joint of the foot, and fractures and dislocations through this area, although not described by Lisfranc, are called Lisfranc's fracture dislocations (Fig. III.22). The eponym arises as a result of Lisfranc's description of a level of amputation through the tarsometatarsal joints, and subsequently this region was given his name.

The injury is usually the result of direct trauma or a lateral rotation injury of the forefoot. As a result, there is commonly lateral and dorsal dislocation of the metatarsals. Medial or divergent dislocations in which the first metatarsal is displaced medially and plantarward and the rest of the metatarsals lateral and dorsal also occur. Dislocation as an isolated injury is rare but is usually associated with fractures of the cunneiform bones and/or the bases of the metatarsals.

Maisonneuve's Fracture

Maisonneuve's fracture is a fracture of the proximal third of the fibula in conjunction with rupture of the distal tibiofibular syndesmosis (Fig. III.23). An associated fracture of the tibia or rupture of the deltoid ligament may be present.

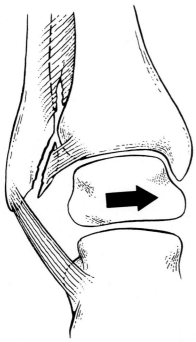

FIG. III.21. Le Fort's fracture.

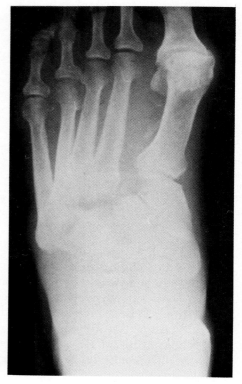

FIG. III.22. Lisfranc's fracture. Fracture dislocation of the tarsal metatarsal joint of the 2nd, 3rd, 4th, and 5th metatarsals.

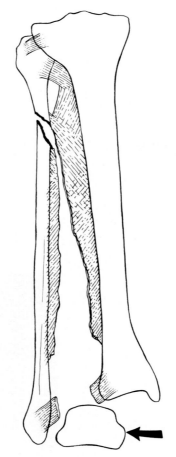

Fig. III.23. Maisonneuve's fracture.

The lesion was described by Maisonneuve in 1840, at which time, based on clinical studies and anatomic dissections, he classified injuries to the fibula caused by internal and external rotation forces.

The lesion that bears his name is caused by an abduction and external rotation force applied to the ankle, which forces the talus laterally against the fibula, initially producing rupture of the inferior tibiofibular syndesmosis. As the force is maintained, the fibula, freed from the tibia, continues to be displaced laterally and posteriorly. The supe-

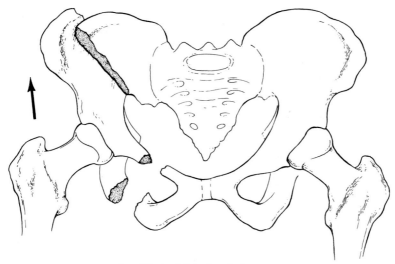

FIG. III.24. Malgaigne's fracture.

rior tibiofibular joint, remaining intact, secures the proximal fibula so that the long lever of the fibula, which further increases the force, produces a fracture of the fibula in its proximal third.

Malgaigne's Fracture

Malgaigne's fracture consists of two vertical fractures involving one side of the pelvic ring, such that one fracture line occurs anterior to the acetabulum and the other posterior to the acetabulum (Fig. III.24).

Malgaigne described this lesion in 1847, prior to the advent of x-ray, to distinguish an entity which clinically resembled a fracture of the neck of the femur. The injury is usually the result of direct trauma which causes a double vertical fracture of the pelvis, with one fracture line extending anterior to the acetabulum, usually through the pubic rami, and the other posterior to the acetabulum, usually through the ilium. Separation of the sacroiliac joint may occur in place of the posterior fracture.

As a result, the hemipelvis is divided into three fragments, with the middle fragment containing the hip joint, completely separated anteriorly and posteriorly. The middle fragment, now completely freed, tends to be displaced, most commonly upward, accompanied by the femur, resulting in changes in the length of the extremity. Other displacements include various inclinations of the middle fragment with the anterior border displaced into the pelvis and the posterior border projecting outward, or the distal aspect depressed inward with flaring of the superior margin.

The result of this fracture is apparent shortening of the lower extremity of approximately ½ inch with the foot more or less everted. This finding, in addition to crepitus elicited by pushing up on the femur or pressing upon the greater trochanter, had caused this fracture frequently to be misdiagnosed as the more common fracture of the neck of the femur. Malgaigne stressed that the distinction between this fracture and one of the femoral neck had to be made through careful measurement of the limb, noting that shortening does not take place in the thigh but that the anterosuperior iliac spine is higher than it should be. Now, of course, radiographic techniques make the differential diagnosis relatively easy.

March Fracture

A march fracture generally refers to a stress or fatigue fracture of the metatarsals. The fracture is the result of repeated relatively trivial trauma to an otherwise normal bone and its name derives from the fact that these fractures are most commonly found in military recruits who are subjected to unaccustomed vigorous activities in the form of marching or hiking. March fractures involve the neck and shaft of the metatarsal, most commonly the second metatarsal. It, however, is not limited just to military personnel, as the unconditioned athlete, the new door-to-door salesman, and the weekend physical fitness enthusiast may all develop march fractures.

At the onset of the patient's symptoms, the x-rays may be normal; however, 2–14 days later, the lesion will appear as a small cortical defect, a fullblown fracture, or periosteal reaction. Serial x-rays afford the best method of diagnosis of this lesion (see "Stress Fractures," page 30).

Monteggia's Fracture

Monteggia's fracture is a fracture of the proximal third of the ulna accompanied by anterior dislocation of the radial head (Fig. III.25). The mechanism of injury is the transmission of a force following a fall on the outstretched hand, through the hand and forearm with the elbow partially flexed.

This injury was described by Giovanni Battista Monteggia in 1814, in his dissertation on dislocations of the head of the radius. At this time, he cited two cases of dislocation of the head of the radius associated with fracture of the proximal ulna and presented a clinical study of a patient who sustained a fracture of the upper third of the ulna, in whom he initially missed the diagnosis of a dislocation of the radial head.

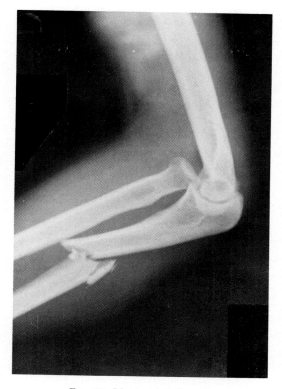

FIG. 25. Monteggia's fracture.

Following routine immobilization for 1 month, the swelling subsided and he then noted the anterior displacement of the head of the radius when the forearm was extended. The prominence was readily reducible with compression of the radial head but recurred again when the pressure was released. Continued treatment was unsatisfactory in maintaining reduction. Monteggia felt that dislocation of the radial head was a lesion he could readily diagnose; however, in this particular case, with the additional pathology of a fractured ulna, the diagnosis eluded him.

Presently, the term Monteggia's fracture has been used to describe fractures of the proximal ulna accompanied by all dislocations of the radial head; however, based on the original presentation, it should probably be reserved only for those with anterior dislocation. Fractures of the proximal ulna with posterior dislocation of the radial head have also been referred to as reverse Monteggia's fractures.

Moore's Fracture

Moore's fracture is a fracture of the distal radius of the Colles' variety associated with fracture of the ulna styloid and dorsal subluxation of the distal ulna (Fig. III.26). In Colles' original description, he did not describe a fracture of the ulna styloid although presently fractures of the distal radius, with or without fracture of the ulna styloid, bear his name.

The lesion was described by E. M. Moore in 1880 (prior to the advent of x-ray) who drew his conclusions by studying the distal ulna in dissected anatomic specimens and clinical patients who had sustained Colles' fractures associated with a compound fracture of the distal ulna.

Moore felt that a fall on the palm of the hand subjects the radius to fracture within 1 inch from the wrist and that subluxation of the ulna accompanied this fracture in more than half the cases. The mechanism of injury is such that once the radius is fractured, it ceases to afford resistance and continuation of the fracture forces then places strain upon

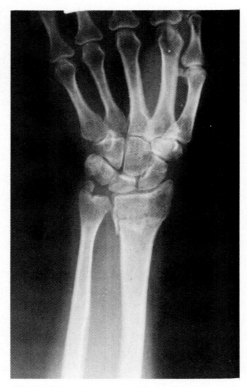

FIG. III.26. Moore's fracture. Note the fracture of the distal ulna. At the present time this lesion would more commonly be referred to as a Colles' fracture.

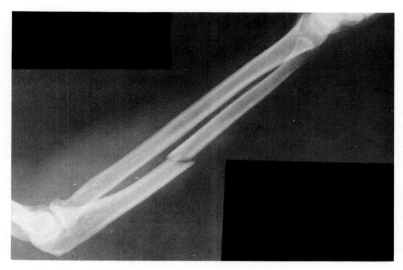

FIG. III.27. Nightstick fracture.

the attachments of the distal aspect of the ulna. The continued strain is then sufficient to rupture the soft tissue connection between the two bones and to cause an avulsion fracture of the styloid process of the ulna. The remaining portion of the distal ulna is displaced dorsally against the dorsal capsule or may rupture its fibers and become caught in it. If the precipitating trauma is severe, the head of the ulna may rupture through all of the soft tissues, including the skin, producing a compound fracture.

Prior to his description, the lesion was believed to be rare. Moore felt that this was a false impression produced by the difficulty in diagnosis of closed lesions and the tremendous force needed to produce compound injuries where the diagnosis was less difficult to demonstrate. To correlate the pathology with clinical findings, he felt that fractures with true silverfork deformity are more apt to be associated with subluxation of the ulna than those in which the hand was carried in more radial direction, the radial deviation implying that the radius was shortened without displacement of the ulna (see "Colles' Fracture," page 298).

Nightstick Fracture

A nightstick fracture is a solitary fracture of the ulna caused by direct trauma when the forearm is raised to parry a blow (Fig. III.27).

Piedmont Fracture

A Piedmont fracture is a closed fracture of the radius at the junction of the middle and distal third, without an associated fracture of the ulna (Fig. III.28).

The lesion was presented in a series of cases from the Piedmont Orthopedic Society of Durham, North Carolina, as an uncommon fracture caused by direct trauma to the forearm. The purpose of the paper was to present the errors in the common method of management of these fractures and to recommend open reduction and secure internal fixation in place of closed reductions which were found to have a high degree of failure.

Pott's Fracture

Pott's fracture, as classically described, is a partial dislocation of the ankle with fracture of the fibula within 2–3 inches above the lateral malleolus and rupture of the medial ligaments of the ankle (Fig. III.29).

Presently Pott's fracture is used to describe bimalleolar fractures, usually those having an avulsion fracture of the medial malleolus caused by an abduction and external rotation injury, although many

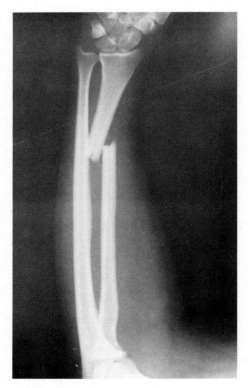

Fig. III.28. Piedmont fracture.

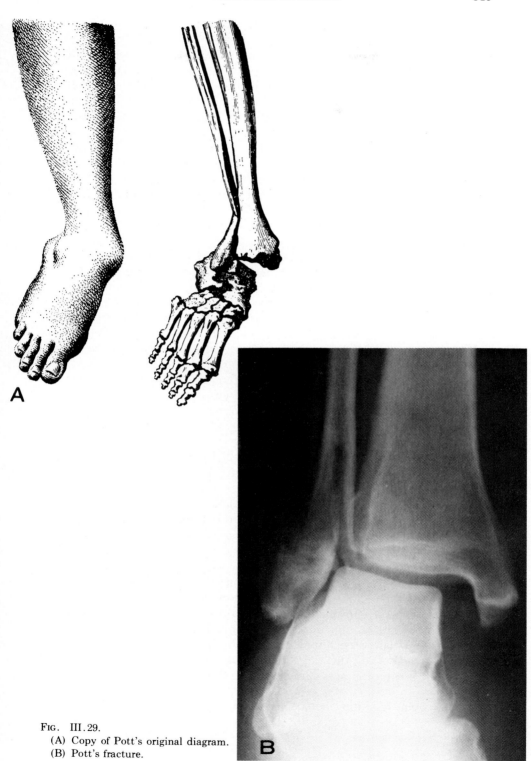

Fig. III.29.
  (A) Copy of Pott's original diagram.
  (B) Pott's fracture.

different fractures of the ankle have been erroneously called Pott's fractures.

The fracture was described by Percival Pott in 1765, at which time he described a fracture of the fibula associated with dislocation of the tibia, which he stated, "is a case which ... gives infinite pain and trouble both to patient and surgeon and very frequently ends in the lameness and disappointment of the former and the disgrace and concern of the latter."

Pott felt that the stability of the ankle is derived from the fibula and that the integrity of the ankle joint depended on the perpendicular relationship of the tibia and talus and the firm connection with the fibula. Any joint disruption which would cause the tibia to be displaced from its perpendicular position on the talus could occur only by rupture of the ligaments which connect the tibia with the talus and os calcis.

He felt that the mechanism of injury is trauma which fractures the fibula within 2–3 inches proximal to its distal end, resulting in the proximal aspect of the distal fragment falling inward toward the tibia and the distal end turned outward and upward (lateral angular displacement of the distal fragment). The ankle joint, now without the support of the fibula, permits medial displacement of the tibia on the talus, leading to rupture of tibiotalar and calcaneal ligaments and resulting in a fracture dislocation of the ankle with the foot being turned outward and upward.

The term, "inverted Pott's fracture," although not described by Pott, is an eponym which, at times, has been used to describe a bimalleolar fracture having an avulsion fracture of the lateral malleolus and a shearing fracture of the medial malleolus (see Fig. II.55B, page 136).

Rolando's Fracture

Rolando's fracture is a Y-shaped intraarticular fracture at the base of the first metacarpal (Fig. III.30).

The fracture was described by Silvio Rolando in 1910, at which time he presented the mechanism of injury and the differential features from a Bennett's fracture. He felt that the dorsal cortex of the first metacarpal exerted stronger resistance to forces applied in the long axis of the bone than did the palmar surface. Therefore, trauma in the longitudinal axis of the metacarpal, if mild, fractured only the palmar surface and produced the oblique fracture of the Bennett's variety. If the force was one of severe magnitude, however, produced by a punch or a fall on the hand with the thumb in the palm, the fracture now extended to involve the dorsal cortex, producing the Y-shaped fracture. He noted that displacement of the large diaphyseal fragment can occur, but rarely does, as in a Bennett's fracture. The fragment usually remains in place.

The eponym, Rolando fracture, has been erroneously used to describe

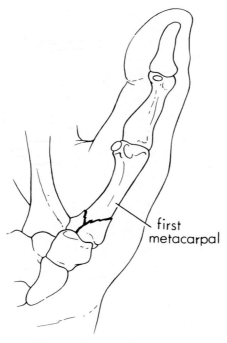

first
metacarpal

FIG. III.30. Rolando's fracture.

transverse fractures through the base of the thumb metacarpal. This
description has, at times, been applied to fractures that have extension
of the transverse fracture into the joint and, at times, has been limited
to just the transverse fractures through the base of the metacarpal.
When the eponym is incorrectly applied to injuries with intraarticular
involvement, the lesion is described as a T-shaped fracture in which a
separate fracture line divides the articular margin into two fragments.

Rolando's fracture has also been referred to as a Bennett's fracture of
the Rolando variety; however, unlike the Bennett's fracture, there is
little tendency toward dislocation (see "Bennett's Fracture," page 289).

Segond's Fracture

Segond's fracture is a fracture of the margin of the lateral tibial condyle and represents an avulsion fracture of the bony insertion of the
tensor fascia lata (iliotibial band). The significance of the lesion rests in
its differential diagnosis, from an avulsion fracture of the tip of the
proximal fibula (Fig. III.31).

Shepherd's Fracture

Shepherd's fracture is a fracture of the lateral tubercle of the posterior process of the talus.

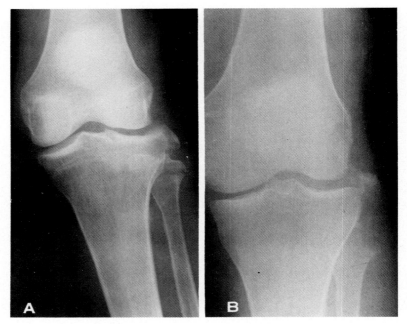

Fig. III.31.
  (A) Segond's fracture.
  (B) Avulsion fracture of the head of the fibula. Note the similarity of the two lesions.

In 1882, Shepherd described what he felt to be a fracture of this region based on multiple anatomic dissections, noting that the lesion
could only be found by dissection, since it caused no deformity and
only vague symptoms. In view of the paucity of symptomatic com-
plaints and clinical findings, Shepherd described what was probably an
os trigonum, and this feeling was held by critics in his time.

Fractures through this region may occur, however. Inasmuch as the
lateral tubercle of the posterior process may form from a separate ossicle (the os trigonum), fusion of this ossicle to the talus, when it occurs, produces a very prominent bony ridge, which, at times, may over-
hand the os calcis. This prominence is susceptible to injury and a fracture through this region may occur and be considered a Shepherd's
fracture (see "Os Trigonum," page 334; see Fig. IV.5B, page 339).

Sideswipe Fracture of the Elbow

A sideswipe fracture is a comminuted fracture of the elbow sustained
by severe direct trauma to the elbow protruding from the window of an
automobile when the upper extremity is resting on the window ledge.

The exposed aspect of the elbow is struck by a vehicle approaching in the opposite direction, or strikes a stationary object. The result is a markedly comminuted fracture of the distal humerus. In addition, the fracture may involve the shaft of the humerus, the olecranon, the shaft of the ulna, and extend to include the head of the radius and coronoid process.

Smith's Fracture

Smith's fracture, as originally described, is a fracture of the distal radius with volar and proximal displacement of the distal fragment, and dorsal displacement of the distal ulna (Fig. III.32).

Presently a Smith's fracture (sometimes referred to as a reverse

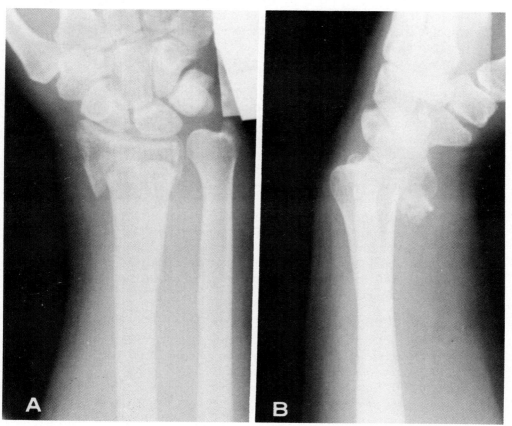

FIG. III.32. (A and B) Smith's fracture—anteroposterior (A) and lateral (B) x-ray.

Colles fracture) is a term applied to fractures of the distal radius in which there is volar displacement of the distal fragment without emphasis placed on the status of the distal ulna. In these instances, the distal ulna may or may not be displaced and the styloid process may be fractured.

The fracture was described by Robert William Smith in 1847 and, in similar fashion to the Colles' fracture, is based on the external characteristics of a clinical deformity rather than radiographically.

The fracture was described as a rare injury produced by a fall on the back of the hand, occurring ½ to 1 inch above the distal radial articulation, the deformity of which resembled a volar dislocation of the carpus. Smith described the deformity as a dorsal prominence produced by the end of the proximal fragment of the radius, accompanied by the distal ulna which has been displaced dorsally and a palmar prominence produced principally by the distal fragment of the radius. The ease of reduction followed by the recurrence of the deformity after release of traction, the presence of crepitus with traction, and the palpable irregular margin of the radius enabled him to distinguish the injury from a carpal dislocation.

Stieda's Fracture

Stieda's fracture is an avulsion fracture of the medial femoral condyle at the origin of the tibial collateral ligament.

The injury was described by Stieda in 1908 but now is usually considered as part of Pellegrini-Stieda's disease of which there are several varieties. The first, or classical type, occurs very rarely and is a radiographic density parallel to and separated from the medial femoral condyle that is noted immediately after an accident, suggesting, and most likely representing, a fracture.

The second type appears as a delayed response resulting in ossification adjacent to the medial femoral condyle at the level where the shaft flares to become the medial condyle. This entity occurs as a result of tearing or shredding of the fibers of the femoral attachments of the tibial collateral ligament and represents ossification within the ligament or hematoma (Fig. III.33).

"Teardrop" Fracture Dislocations of the Cervical Spine

A "teardrop" fracture dislocation or an acute flexion fracture dislocation of the cervical spine is a compression fracture of the body of a cervical vertebra, resulting in compression of the anterior aspect of the involved body and separation of a fragment of bone. The mechanism of injury is a severe hyperflexion compression force which causes bursting of the body, separation, and anterior and inferior displacement of a triangular shaped fragment from the anteroinferior margin of the involved

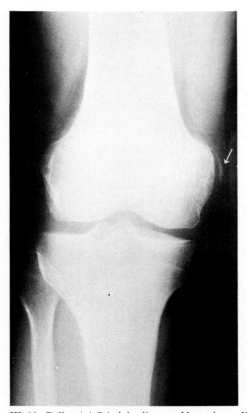

FIG. III.33. Pellegrini-Stieda's disease. Note the radiodensity adjacent to the medial femoral condyle. An
acute avulsion fracture in this area would be called a
Stieda's fracture.

vertebral body. Simultaneously the posteroinferior margin of the same vertebral body is displaced posteriorly into the spinal canal (Fig. III.34).

The name is derived from the appearance of the fracture, which looks like a drop of water dripping from the vertebral body. The significance of this injury rests in its potential danger to the spinal cord as the posterior displacement of the inferior margin of the vertebra into the spinal canal often causes compression or destruction of the anterior portion of the cervical spinal cord.

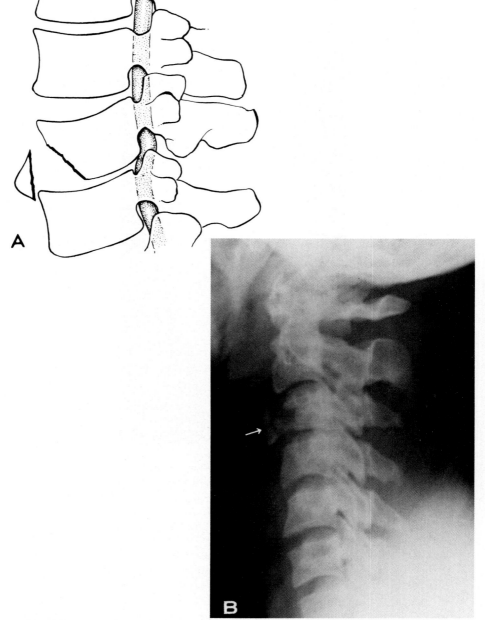

Fig. III.34. Teardrop fracture.
    (A) Note how the spinal cord may be compressed by the posteroinferior aspect of the vertebrae.
    (B) Radiograph of a teardrop fracture of the third cervical vetebra.

Thurston Holland's Fragment

Thurston Holland's fragment is the triangular metaphyseal fragment that accompanies the epiphysis in an epiphyseal separation (Fig. III.35).

The lesion was described by Thurston Holland in 1929 in order to radiographically identify epiphyseal injuries when the epiphysis had spontaneously reduced or had been reduced by the physician. He based his paper on studies of the distal radius and felt that this was the most common site of involvement. He believed that an isolated epiphyseal fracture, that is, one in which the fracture line extends only through the cartilage plate between the epiphysis and the metaphysis, is rare (Salter-Harris Type I), noting that most commonly there is metaphyseal injury as well. The lesion consists of a segment of metaphysis of variable size which accompanies the epiphysis and is displaced in the same direction as the epiphysis.

Thus in injuries in which there was an isolated epiphyseal separation following spontaneous reduction or reduction by a surgeon, no radiographic evidence would be present that injury had taken place. In fractures in which a metaphyseal fragment was present, however, positive evidence of epiphyseal injury now existed, and the diagnosis of epiphyseal injury could be made even if the epiphysis had returned to its normal anatomic position at the time of x-ray. Although he felt that the distal radius was most commonly involved, he noted that the lesion also occurs in displacement of the epiphyses of other bones.

Tillaux's Fracture

Tillaux's fracture presently is considered to be a fracture involving the distal lateral articular surface of the tibia in which the fracture line runs vertically from the distal articular surface upward to the lateral cortex. The fracture fragment may be small or large, and may involve the anterior or posterior tubercle, or both (Fig. III.36). As originally described by Tillaux, however, the lesion was not an isolated fracture but the component of a more complicated fracture which contained several fragments.

The fracture was first described by Sir Astley Cooper in 1822 and, after a period of 50 years, in 1872, Gosselin again described the pathology in presenting a thesis on Tillaux's work in this area, entitled, "The Clinical and Experimental Research of Fractures of the Malleoli." At that time, the lesion was described as the result of a rotation injury where force initially fractured the lateral malleolus and, continuing, produced an avulsion fracture of the tibia by the pull of the inferior tibiofibular ligament at its insertion if the ligament itself did not first rupture. Tillaux, in 1890, subsequently modified his concept of the mechanics of this fracture, and described it as occurring as the result of the foot being turned outward (forced abduction-pronation). This injury

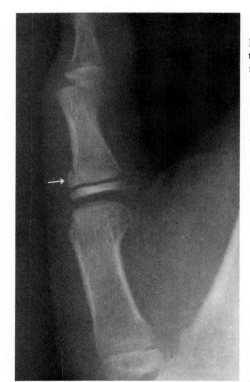

FIG. III.35. Thurston Holland fragment. Note that, although the epiphysis is reduced, the metaphyseal fragment is still visible.

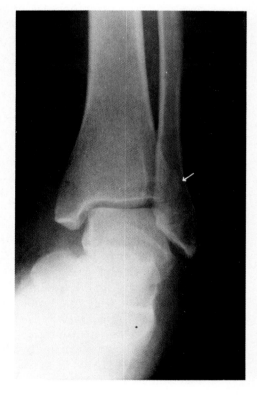

FIG. III.36. Tillaux's fracture.

produced three fragments. Initially, there was fracture of the medial malleolus. As the force was continued, diastasis of the distal tibiofibular syndesmosis occurred with an avulsion fracture of the tibia at the insertion of the distal tibiofibular ligament, followed by a fracture of the lateral malleolus 6–7 cm. proximal to its distal end (Fig. III.37). Although Tillaux did not specifically mention which tubercles were involved, Souligaux, a pupil of Tillaux, published two diagrams by Tillaux demonstrating fragments corresponding to both the anterior and posterior tubercles.

Torus Fracture

A torus fracture is an incomplete fracture with buckling of one cortex. The fracture occurs predominantly in children and usually from a fall on the outstretched hand (see "Torus Fracture," page 52; see Fig. I.35, page 54).

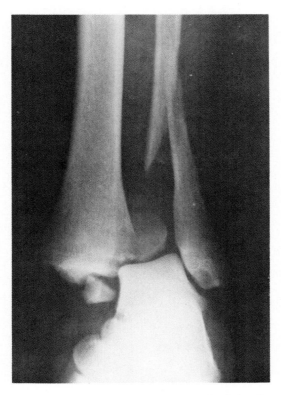

Fig. III.37. Tillaux's fracture composed of the three fragments described by Tillaux.

Wagon Wheel Fracture

A wagon wheel fracture refers to a separation of the distal femoral epiphysis (Fig. III.38). The terminology was based upon the mechanism of injury, wherein legs in many cases were caught in the spokes of a revolving wagon wheel.

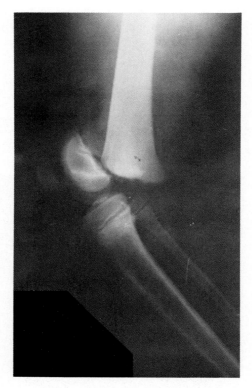

FIG. III.38. Wagon wheel fracture.

PART FOUR

FRACTURES THAT ARE NOT FRACTURES

In the inspection of radiographs, many features may frequently be erroneously interpreted as a fracture. These include most commonly, secondary centers of ossification and accessory bones which have not fused to the main bone, epiphyses before the termination of growth, and, at times, large vascular foramina.

This section is an attempt to demonstrate some of the more common radiologic entities which may lead the unwary into the mistaken diagnosis of a fracture.

ACCESSORY BONES

Accessory bones are separate centers of ossification which are located adjacent to and belong to a particular parent bone. These centers, over a period of time, may obtain or fail to achieve bony union with the parent bone. In the latter situation, they remain as separate ossicles attached by fibrous or cartilaginous bonds. If bony fusion of an accessory bone does occur, it generally causes the parent bone to be enlarged with a bony prominence, essentially corresponding to the size of the extra ossicle.

Accessory bones are found frequently in the skeleton and most commonly in the foot.

Accessory bones present difficulty in the interpretation of fractures, as unfused accessory bones may simulate fractures. Fractures through a fused prominence, in contrast, may be misinterpreted as an unfused accessory bone. Roentgenographic differentiation may be assisted by noting that accessory bones have smooth, rounded borders surrounded by cortical bone and are usually bilateral. Recent fractures, however, have irregular opposing surfaces which are relatively more lucent than the denser cortical appearance and will not be present in the opposite extremity.

In an attempt to avoid mistaken diagnoses, some of the more common accessory bones will be presented.

Accessory Bones of the Ankle and Foot

Besides the bones which are normally present in the foot, there are many accessory bones, each originating from a separate center of ossification (Fig. IV.1).

Radiographic examination of a foot with separate ossicles may give the impression of a fracture, and thus one must be aware of their presence. This is especially so when a recently injured foot with the symptomatology of a fracture is x-rayed.

Os Subtibiale and Os Subfibulare

The os subtibiale is a separate ossification center, located just below the tip of the medial malleolus, which remains as a discrete ossicle. There are varying opinions as to the etiology of the os subtibiale. Between the 6th and 12th years of life, a separate ossification center can be present at the tip of the medial malleolus. This center has been referred to, by some, as the os subtibiale. Other authorities felt that this ossification center is not, and should be differentiated from, the os subtibiale and classified this area as an accessory epiphysis for the medial malleolus (Fig. IV.2). Inasmuch as fusion of this center would not en-

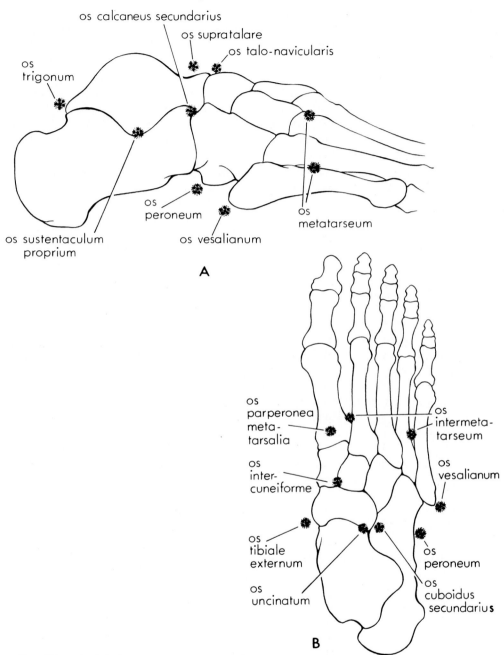

FIG. IV.1. (A and B) Anteroposterior and lateral views indicating the sites of the accessory bones of the foot. These bones may exist separately or be united to the parent bones.

large the parent bone as would an extra ossicle, it would appear that it is an accessory epiphysis and the os subtibiale is an independent structure. A third concept is that the os subtibiale is calcification in the deltoid ligament secondary to trauma or an avulsion fracture of the medial malleolus.

Corresponding to the os subtibiale, the os subfibulare is a separate center for the tip of the lateral malleolus.

These areas (os subtibiale and os subfibulare) vary from small rounded ossicles to fairly large triangular fragments and are best seen on the anteroposterior views of the ankle joint. Despite the etiology of these bony areas, differentiation must be made from fractures of the medial and lateral malleoli (Fig. IV.3).

Os Tibiale Externum (Accessory Navicular)

The os tibiale externum (accessory navicular) is perhaps the most common of the accessory bones of the foot, and appears between the 10th and 12th years of life as an ossicle on the medial aspect of the tarsal navicular. If the accessory bone fuses to the navicular, it forms a large tuberosity on the medial aspect of the tarsal navicular which curves slightly posteriorly about the talus. As this ossicle serves for the insertion of the tibialis posterior, a fused accessory navicular is predisposed to avulsion fractures which may result from an abduction injury to the foot.

Thus differentiation must be made between an os tibiale externum and an avulsion fracture through the tuberosity of the tarsal navicular (Fig. IV.4). This differentiation may be assisted by noting that, with an os tibiale externum, the border opposing the navicular is smooth with a cortical margin, shows no sharp irregularities, and is usually bilateral. In a fresh fracture, the fracture line is irregular, without smooth borders, and is not found bilaterally.

Os Trigonum

Posteriorly, the talus is projected into a posterior process which consists of a medial and lateral tubercle located on either side of a sulcus, grooved by the tendon of the flexor hallucis longus.

The lateral tubercle, at times, forms from a separate center of ossification which is called the os trigonum. This ossicle may vary in size, from a small bony element to a large mass. With fusion of the os trigonum to the talus, the lateral tubercle will be enlarged and project posteriorly, and at times, may overhang the os calcis. With failure of fusion of this accessory bone to the main body of the talus, the os trigonum

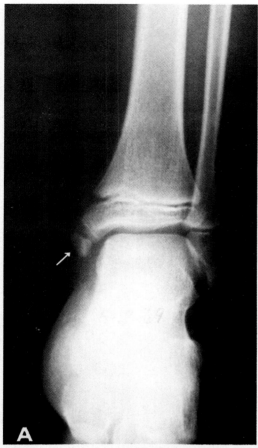

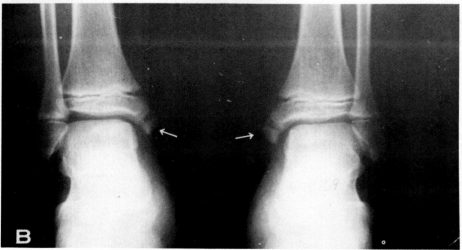

FIG. IV.2.

(A) Accessory apophysis in a child which appears like a fracture of the medial malleolus.

(B) Comparative x-ray shows the same bony structure present in the opposite extremity.

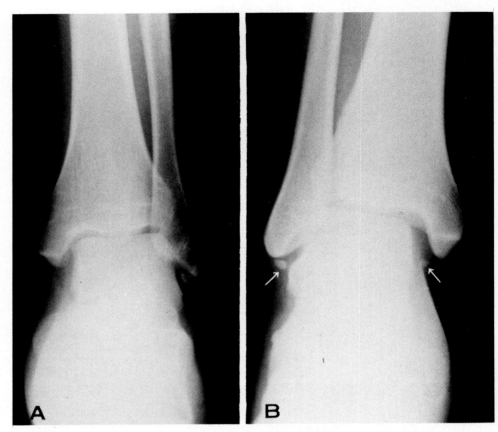

Fɪɢ. IV.3.

(A) Os subfibulare. Note that the extra ossicle appears as an avulsion fracture of the lateral malleolus; however, the borders are smooth, and one can delineate the complete appearance of the lateral malleolus.

(B) Radiograph demonstrating extra ossicles beneath the tibia and the fibula, probably representing an os subtibiale and an os subfibulare inasmuch as both malleoli appear intact. Since there is widening of the mortise however, it may be argued that there is ossification in the deltoid ligament or an old avulsion fracture of the medial malleolus.

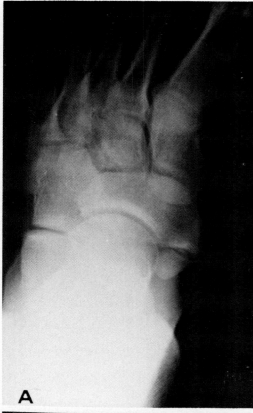

Fig. IV.4. Os tibiale externum (accessory navicular).

(A) Note the enlarged size of the tarsal navicular which is curving slightly posteriorly about the talus. A radiolucent line divides the prominent tuberosity which gives the appearance of a fracture.

(B) Comparative x-ray reveals the symmetrical appearance of the navicular and the bilateral nature of the defect.

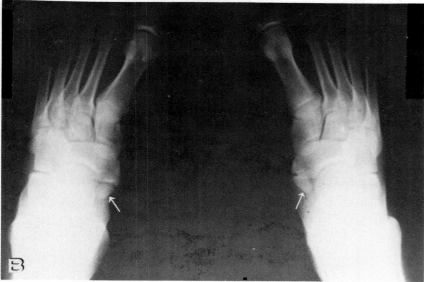

will remain as a separate ossicle. This feature may simulate a fracture on x-ray (Fig. IV.5) and, as previously noted in this book, this entity was described by Shepherd (see "Shepherd's Fracture," page 321). Thus several factors may be considered: that of an ununited os trigonum appearing as a fracture, or a true fracture through a fused trigonal process being misinterpreted as an os trigonum. Differentiation may be assisted by noting that an os trigonum will be somewhat rounded and have smooth opposing borders bounded by cortical bone, as opposed to a fresh fracture through a trigonal process which would be irregular in shape (mainly triangular) with an irregular fracture line and without dense opposing surfaces.

Os Vesalianum (Os Versale)

The os vesalianum is an accessory center of ossification located just proximal and lateral to the base of the fifth metatarsal (Fig. IV.6). This center may fail to fuse with the parent bone and, if so, may be confused with an avulsion fracture of the base of the fifth metatarsal, or the epiphysis at the base of the fifth metatarsal. Distinction may be made by noting the complete shape of the ossicle and the complete shape of the fifth metatarsal, in addition to the other general distinguishing features of accessory bones and fractures noted earlier (See "Epiphysis of the Fifth Metatarsal," page 356).

Although rare, an os vesalianum may be present in the hand, proximal to the base of the fifth metacarpal.

Calcaneus Secundarius

The calcaneus secundarius is a small, irregular ossicle located at the upper anterior aspect of the os calcis, adjacent to the articulations with the astragalus and the navicular. Its shape is variable as is its size. It may be extremely difficult to differentiate the secondary calcaneus from fractures of the superior articulation of the calcaneus (Fig. IV.7). Comparative x-rays as well as evaluation of the apposing surfaces, as previously described, may assist in the diagnosis. At times, it may be necessary to have serial x-rays over an extended period of time to demonstrate fracture healing before the diagnosis can be made.

Os Supranaviculare—Piries Bone (Dorsal Talonavicular Ossicle)

The os supranaviculare is an ossicle located in the superior talonavicular joint, anterior to the superior surface of the talus and posterior to the superior surface of the navicular. It is relatively common, seen on

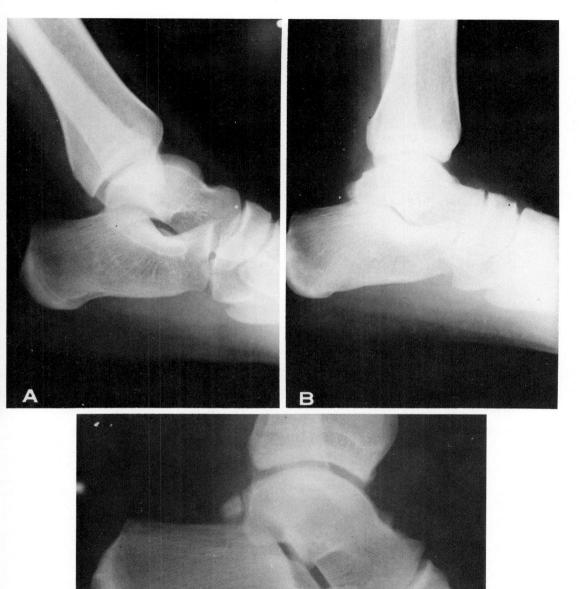

FIG. IV.5. Os trigonum.

(A) Normal talus.

(B) Normal talus with an enlarged posterior lateral tubercle, probably due to a fused os trigonum.

(C) The enlarged posterior lateral tubercle of the talus has a lucent line dividing the prominence, which gives the appearance of a fracture. On closer inspection, the apposing borders appear smooth and regular with evidence of subchondral bone. This patient had no history of trauma and was asymptomatic in this region. The x-ray was for problems elsewhere in the foot.

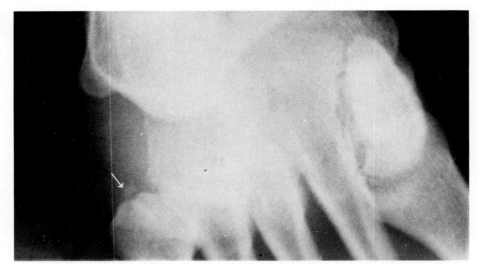

FIG. IV.6. Os versale. A small ossicle is present proximal to the base of the fifth metatarsal.

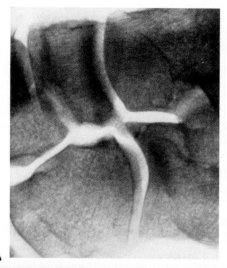

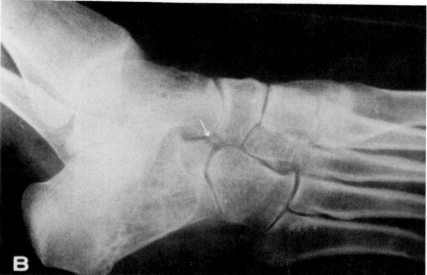

FIG. IV.7.

(A) Calcaneus secundarius. Note the extra ossicle and the complete appearance of the anterior aspect of the os calcis. (From A. Kohler and E. A. Zimmer: *Borderlands of the Normal and Early Pathologic in Skeletal Roentgenology*, p. 491, Grune & Stratton, New York, 1968.)

(B) Defect anterior to the os calcis represents a fracture of the anterior aspect of the os calcis. Note the irregular lucent fracture line and absence of sclerotic margins and cortical surfaces.

lateral radiographs, and may be mistaken for a fracture of the navicular or talus (Fig. IV.8).

Os Peroneum (Peroneal Sesamoid)

The os peroneum is a sesamoid located in the tendon of the peroneus longus on the plantar aspect of the foot between the os calcis and cuboid (Fig. IV.9). Occasionally there may be two or three separate ossicles representing a bipartite or tripartite sesamoid. Also, great variation may exist in the size and shape of the ossicle. The peroneal sesamoid is frequently bilateral and is most readily noted on lateral or oblique views. The peroneal sesamoid may simulate a fracture; however, it usually offers no trouble in diagnosis.

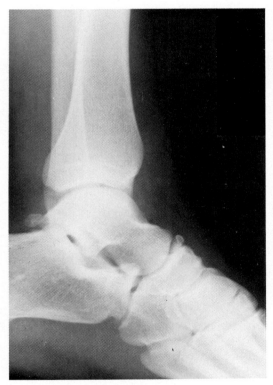

Fig. IV.8. Os supranaviculare. An extra ossicle is present which appears as a fracture of the navicular. The completeness of each structure can be seen as well as the smooth apposing borders. An os trigonum is also present.

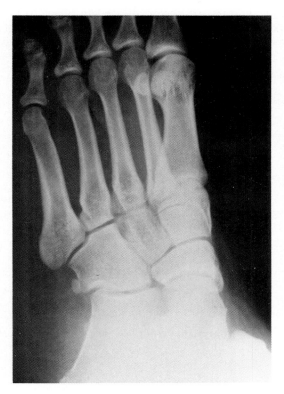

FIG. IV.9. Os peroneum. Note the small, rounded density adjacent to the cuboid. Although on occasion it may stimulate a fracture, it usually offers no trouble in diagnosis.

Less Common Accessory Bones of the Foot That May Simulate Fractures

Besides those already mentioned, additional ossicles are found on radiographic examination of the foot.

Os Intermetatarseum

The os intermetatarseum is a small ossicle in the form of a tiny rudimentary metatarsal found between the proximal ends of the first and second metatarsals. At times, because of overlapping shadows, it may appear as a fracture of the first metatarsal. Additional views will demonstrate the completeness of the accessory ossicle (Fig. IV.10).

Os Intercuneiform

The os intercuneiform is a small ossicle situated on the dorsum of the foot between the proximal aspect of the first and second cuneiform bones.

Os Sustentaculare

This is a wedge-shaped ossicle that comprises the upper posterior end of the sustentaculum tali. The ossicle usually is triangular in shape although it may be round and variable in size.

Os Uncinatum

The os uncinatum is a small ossicle on the plantar aspect of the lateral cuneiform.

Cuboideum Secundarium (Cuboides Secundarius)

This is another rare bone which is located between the navicular, talus, and cuboid.

Os Supratalare

The os supratalare is a small rounded bone found just above the head of the talus and is seen only in lateral views of the foot. It should not be confused with the os supranaviculare, which lies between the talus and the navicular, and must be differentiated from an avulsion fracture of the talus (Fig. IV.11).

Accessory Bones of the Pelvis

Os Acetabuli

The os acetabuli, to the anatomist, is the largest ossicle of a group of ossicles which normally forms the roof of the acetabulum, along with the other three major components of the innominate bone. Radiographically it appears as an ossification center located within the superior rim of the acetabulum.

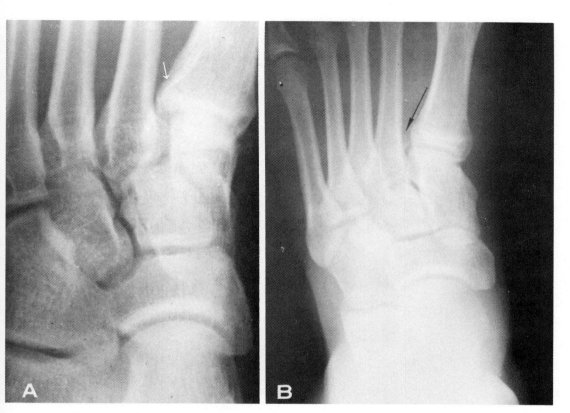

Fig. IV.10. Os intermetatarsum.

(A) A lucent line is present laterally at the base of the first metatarsal which gives the appearance of a nondisplaced fracture.

(B) Additional view demonstrates the ossicle between the proximal ends of the first and second metatarsals.

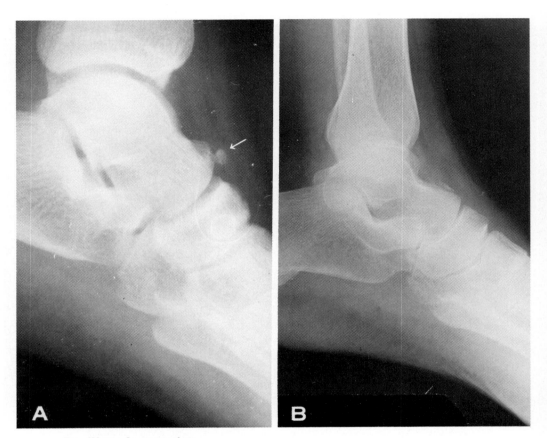

FIG. IV.11. Os supratalare.
(A) Note that the ossicle is rounded, smooth, with cortical margins, and has produced no defect in the talus, as opposed to an avulsion fracture, as shown in (B).
(B) Avulsion fracture. Note that the apposing borders show no cortical margins and the defect in the talus is clearly visible.

Frequently an ossicle is present adjacent to the superior rim or located in the posterior or superior rim of the acetabulum. Although commonly referred to as the os acetabuli by the radiologist, it should not be confused with the anatomist's os acetabuli. This small ossicle is, at times, misinterpreted as an avulsion fracture; however, its smooth border and the complete shape of the acetabulum should assist in the diagnosis (Fig. IV.12).

Accessory Bones of the Wrist and Hand

Accessory bones are present in the upper extremity but are less common than those of the foot. They are located primarily at the wrist and shoulder.

Os Triangulare and Radiale Externum

The os triangulare is an accessory bone located just below the ulna styloid, between it and the triangular (triquetrum) bone. Opinions vary as to the interpretation of this ossicle. In some cases, it has been classified as an old avulsion fracture of the ulna styloid, and others believe it to be soft tissue calcification. It has also been reported to be present bilaterally without preexisting history of trauma and, therefore, probably represents an independent ossicle. In any case, if it is truly an accessory ossicle, it must be differentiated from a recent or ununited fracture of the ulna styloid. Differentiation may be difficult, especially in the presence of an old distal radial or carpal fracture or dislocation. This differentiation from a fracture of the ulna styloid may be assisted by noting the length and completeness of the ulna styloid. If the styloid process is of normal contour and no defects are present indicating the location of an avulsed fragment, the area of ossification probably represents an accessory ossicle. At this point, however, it should be noted that at times the ulna styloid may arise from a separate center of ossification and failure of fusion of this center would lead to disruption of the normal contour of the styloid. In a recent fracture, the fracture line will be found dividing the ulna styloid without the presence of dense apposing surfaces (Fig. IV.13). Comparative x-rays can assist in the diagnosis if the condition is found to be bilateral.

The radiale externum is a rare small ossicle lying just distal to the styloid process of the radius.

Navicular Os Centrale

In the lower primates, there is an extra free bone which, in man, fuses to the navicular in the 3rd month of fetal life. On rare occasions it may remain free, lying between the navicular, capitate, and lesser multangular, and appear as a fracture.

Other rare accessory ossicles are present at the wrist and can be found adjacent to most of the carpal bones.

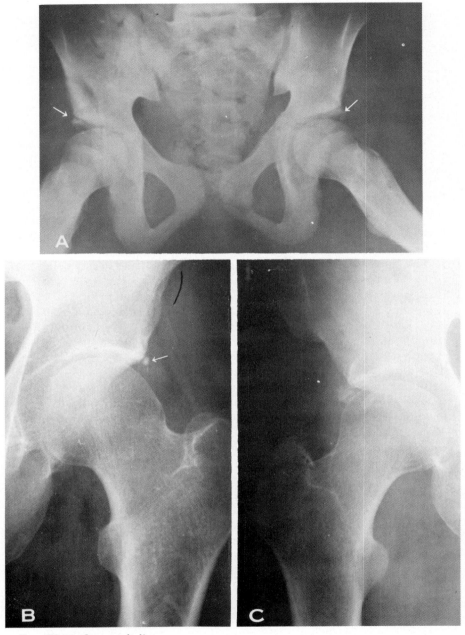

FIG. IV.12. Os acetabuli.

(A) Bilateral true os acetabuli.

(B) The small density adjacent to the superior margin of the acetabulum may appear as an avulsion fracture. The borders, however, are smooth and the structure of the acetabulum complete. Although not truly the os acetabuli, it is frequently referred to as such.

(C) Similar lesion of larger size. Note that the bony element lies outside of the rim of the acetabulum.

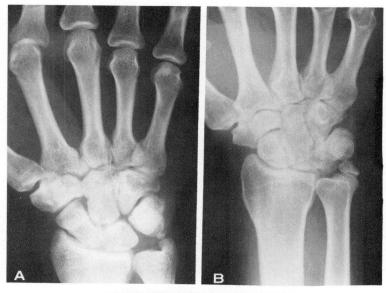

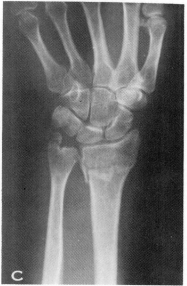

Fig. IV.13. Os triangulare.

(A) A small ossicle is located distal to the ulna styloid. The ulna styloid appears complete in shape and the apposing surfaces have evidence of subchondral bone.

(B) Difficulty arises in cases where there is an old injury to the wrist. In this case, there was an old dislocation of the lunate. The apposing surfaces of the distal ulna are smooth and contain cortical margins. The injury probably represents a nonunion of the ulna styloid, inasmuch as the shape of the fragment would complete the design of a normal styloid. Failure of fusion of a separate ulna styloid ossification center can also be considered.

(C) Recent fracture. Note the borders are lucent and without sclerotic margins.

Accessory Bones of the Shoulder

Os Acromiale

During the 15th to 18th years, several ossification centers develop at the lateral end of the acromion which first fuse with each other and then with the scapula. Persistence of this ossification center is called the os acromiale. The os acromiale is variable in size and shape and is usually bilateral.

At times, a small secondary or accessory os acromiale may be present and found directly above the greater tuberosity of the humerus. This ossicle is separated from the acromion by approximately 1 cm, and is usually somewhat circular in shape.

Persistence of the os acromiale may give the appearance of a fracture of the acromion; however, inasmuch as it is usually bilateral, the diagnosis can be made.

The accessory os acromiale can appear as an avulsion fracture and also must be differentiated from a calcific subacromial tendonitis.

EPIPHYSES

Apophysis (Epiphysis) of the Os Calcis

The apophysis of the calcaneus is a normal secondary center of ossification for the development of the tuberosity of the os calcis. It develops between 5 and 12 years of age, from one or more ossification centers, and fuses to the body of the os calcis at about 17 years of age. Prior to union, the appearance of the epiphyseal line may be mistaken for a fracture because of its irregular border, and/or because of the multiple ossification centers which give the epiphysis a segmental comminuted appearance, the apophysis itself may appear to be fractured. Comparative x-rays will help to assist in establishing the diagnosis (Fig. IV.14).

The apophyses of the tuberosity of the os calcis are also characterized by a marked radiodensity. This increased radiodensity has been mistakenly interpreted as avascular necrosis or an apophysitis (Sever's disease). Although pain and tenderness may be present for varying periods of time, the diagnosis of Sever's disease is a clinical one as the increased radiodensity is present in the heels of healthy children.

Epiphyses of the Hand in Children

The epiphyses of the metacarpals and phalanges present variations which, at times, produce mistaken diagnoses in the interpretation of radiographs. Normally, the epiphyses of the phalanges of the thumb, index, middle, ring, and small fingers are located at the proximal end or base of the bone. The epiphyses of the metacarpals, however, are

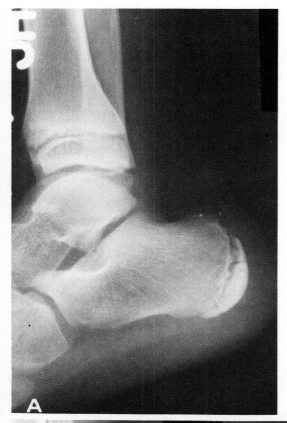

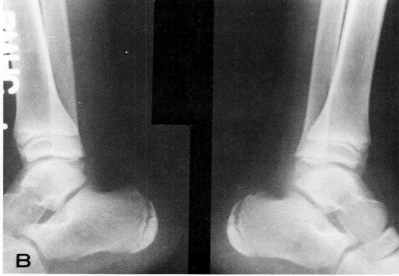

Fig. IV.14.

(A) Apophysis of the os calcis. The irregular margin of the epiphyseal line of the tuberosity of the os calcis and the segmental appearance of the epiphysis itself give the appearance of a fracture of the tuberosity of the os calcis.

(B) Comparative x-rays demonstrate the similar appearance of the apophysis of the opposite extremity. One can also note the increased radiodensity of the calcaneal apophysis, suggesting avascular necrosis.

located distally at the heads with the exception of the metacarpal of the thumb which, like the phalanges, has its epiphysis at the base. This variation may lead to a mistaken diagnosis of a fracture at the base of the first metacarpal, and, conversely, fracture through the head of the first metacarpal may be interpreted by the unwary as a normal epiphysis. Similar mistakes can also be made in the interpretation of fractures of the other metacarpals and phalanges (Fig. IV.15).

At times, an epiphyseal ossification center is present distally in the first metacarpal, or a proximal epiphysis may be seen on the second or fifth metacarpal. These areas develop earlier than do normal epiphyses, increase rapidly in size, and exhibit early closure. Comparative x-rays will assist in proper evaluation.

Epiphysis of the Olecranon and Patella Cubiti

The epiphysis for the olecranon is a separate ossification center which begins to ossify between the ages of 8 and 10 years, fuses at about 16 years of age, and varies greatly in individual appearance. It sometimes contains two centers of ossification, with the initial ossification center usually located at the center of the olecranon and the second center located more proximally at the tip of the olecranon. Gradually the separate centers fuse with each other and, at approximately 16–20 years of age, the ossification centers of the olecranon fuse with the shaft of the ulna. At the time of, or prior to, fusion, the olecranon epiphysis may be misinterpreted as a fracture (Fig. IV.16).

Several features may assist in differentiating the epiphysis from a fracture. Although in both the shape of the olecranon is complete, epiphyses have smooth adjacent surfaces with dense subchondral margins. As the development of the epiphyses are usually bilaterally symmetrical, x-ray examination of the opposite elbow will show a similar pattern. For those cases where the diagnosis is still uncertain, serial x-ray studies will reveal the presence or absence of fracture healing.

The epiphysis of the olecranon should not be confused with patella cubiti which is a bony center that forms in the region of the olecranon (Fig. IV.17). Opinions as to the exact nature of the ossification vary, some feel that it is a large sesamoid which develops in the triceps tendon near the elbow and simulates the appearance of the patella, while others contend that it is an example of either osteochondritis dissecans or calcification of the tendon of the triceps muscle. The condition is generally bilateral and should be differentiated from the olecranon epiphysis and fractures of the olecranon.

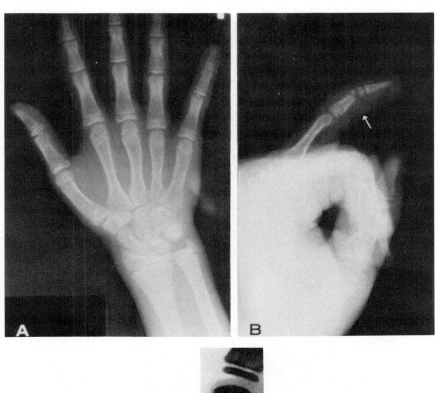

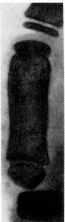

Fig. IV.15.

(A) Location of the epiphyses of the normal hand in a child. Note the variation in the first metacarpal as compared to the other metacarpals.

(B) Transverse fracture of the tip of the middle phalanx which gives the appearance of an epiphyseal separation. Note the proximity of the epiphysis at the base of the distal phalanx.

(C) Accessory epiphysis at the distal aspect of the thumb metacarpal. (From A. Kohler and E. A. Zimmer: *Borderlands of the Normal and Early Pathologic in Skeletal Roentgenology*, p. 80, Grune Stratton, New York, 1968.)

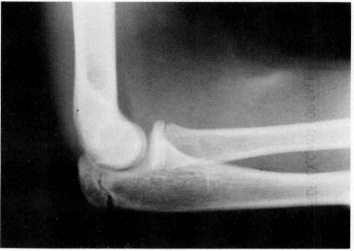

FIG. IV. 16. Epiphysis of the olecranon. The epiphysis of the olecranon is a separate center of ossification which, prior to fusion, may appear as a fracture. Note the smooth adjacent surfaces and the minimal separation. The epiphysis of the head of the radius is still present. All of these factors may assist in the diagnosis.

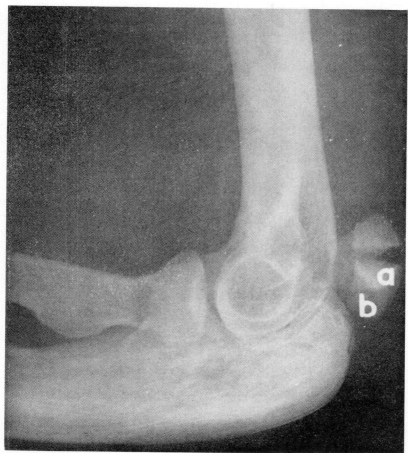

Fig. IV.17. Patella cubiti present in the triceps tendon which has a similar appearance to the patella at the knee. Note the presence of a transverse fracture. (From A. de Lorimier, H. G. Moehring, and J. R. Hannon: *Clinical Radiology*, Vol. 1, p. 111, Charles C Thomas, Springfield, Ill., 1954.)

Epiphysis of the Base of the Fifth Metatarsal

The proximal aspect of the fifth metatarsal develops from a separate epiphysis at about age 13 and unites shortly thereafter; however, it may remain ununited throughout life. This epiphysis may be mistaken for an avulsion fracture of the base of the fifth metatarsal as the opposing margins are irregular and often projected obliquely in such a manner to give the appearance of an avulsed fragment of bone. In addition, multiple nuclei may be present which appear to make the epiphysis look fragmented and comminuted.

Avulsion fractures in this location are common and occur as the result of contraction of the peroneus brevis, usually following a severe inversion injury.

Another entity which appears in this region is the os vesalianum which is an accessory center of ossification located just proximal and lateral to the base of the fifth metatarsal (see "Os vesalianum," page 338). This center may fail to fuse and may be confused with an avulsion fracture of the base of the fifth metatarsal or the epiphysis of this region.

Thus at the base of the fifth metatarsal there are three entities to be differentiated: the os vesalianum (which is a separate ossicle), the epiphysis at the base of the fifth metatarsal, and an avulsion fracture (Fig. IV.18).

The differential diagnosis may be accomplished by critical analysis. The os vesalianum is located adjacent to the base of the fifth metatarsal and the outline of each forms a complete bone. In an avulsion fracture, the fracture surfaces are irregular, with the fracture line usually *transverse* to the long axis of the bone, whereas the epiphyseal line at the base of the fifth metatarsal is *oblique* to the long axis of the bone and is generally bilateral.

Proximal Humeral Epiphysis

The proximal humeral epiphysis develops from three centers of ossification, one for the head and one each for the tuberosities. The tuberosities unite with the capital epiphysis to form a single center at age 5–8 years. In the later stages of a child's growth and development, the epiphyseal line at the proximal humerus may simulate a fracture of the surgical neck (Fig. IV.19). This misinterpretation occurs because of the undulating appearance of the epiphyseal plate in the older child, which in the younger child and at most other locations, is usually relatively straight and transverse. Comparative x-rays and views in other projections will help differentiate the two conditions.

Epiphyses of the Vertebrae

Epiphyseal lines are also present in the vertebrae and may remain ununited throughout life, causing the erroneous interpretation of a fracture.

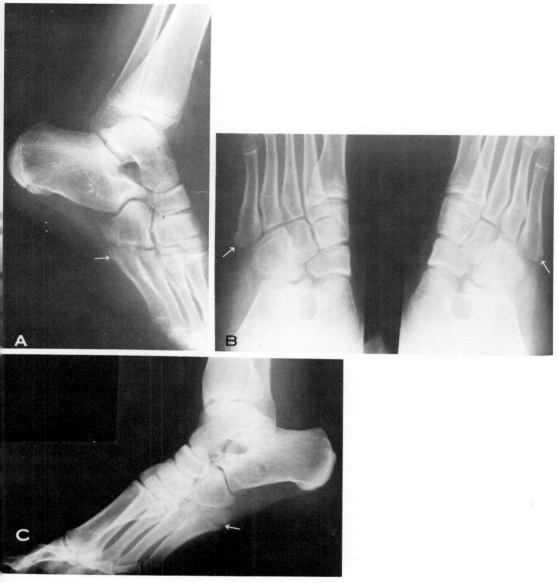

FIG. IV.18. Epiphysis and fracture at the base of the fifth metatarsal.

(A) Epiphysis at the base of the fifth metatarsal can give the appearance of an oblique fracture.

(B) Comparative x-ray reveals the bilateral presence of the epiphysis.

(C) True fracture of the base of the fifth metatarsal. In fractures, the fracture line is usually transverse to the long axis of the bone.

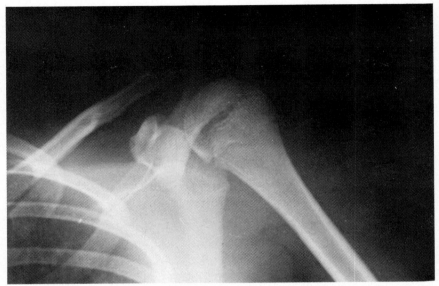

Fig. IV.19. Proximal humeral epiphysis. In the older child, the irregular shape of the epiphyseal line of the proximal humeral epiphysis may simulate a fracture.

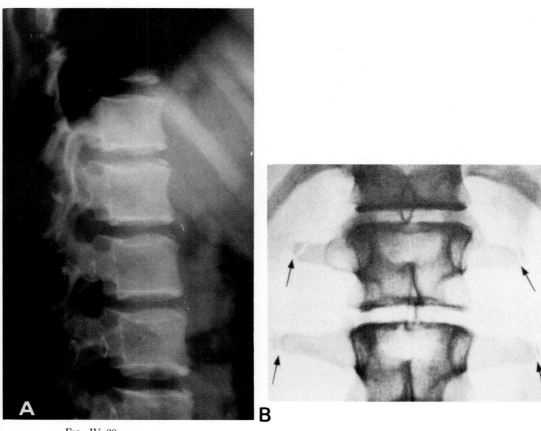

Fig. IV.20.

(A) Epiphyses of vertebrae. The epiphyseal line at the anterior superior and inferior aspect of the vertebral bodies may appear as fractures. Their position and multiple areas involved, however, assist in diagnosis.

(B) Epiphyses of the transverse processes of vertebrae may appear as fractures. (From P. F. Matzen and H. K. Fleissner: *Orthopedic Roentgen Atlas*, p. 20. Grune & Stratton, New York, 1970.

The areas involved are the anterosuperior and anteroinferior margins of the vertebral bodies and the ends of the transverse and spinous processes, suggesting avulsion fractures through these areas (Fig. IV.20).

Evaluation may be difficult, especially in the vertebral bodies and spinous processes as comparative x-rays would not be available. A strong index of suspicion is essential.

In the body of the vertebra, the location of the epiphyses may be helpful inasmuch as they are located just superior or inferior to the body without much anterior displacement. The appearance of multiple centers can also contribute to the differentiation.

JUXTAARTICULAR CALCIFICATION

Calcium deposition at the insertion of the tendons may give the appearance of an avulsion fracture. These calcified foci, however, exhibit no evidence of bone trabeculae, being amorphous or, at times, granular in structure. Furthermore, examination of the contour of the adjacent bone reveals no defect to correspond to the avulsed appearing fragment (Fig. IV.21).

MULTIPARTITE CONDITIONS

Multipartite Patella

The patella is a large sesamoid bone which develops in the tendon of the quadriceps muscle. Ossification of the patella occurs at about 2½ years of age in the female and 3 years of age in the male, generally from a single center of ossification. At times, two or more centers of ossification are present which, on occasion, fail to fuse and remain as separate components. Routine x-rays following a fall will disclose the previously asymptomatic abnormality which may be misinterpreted as a fracture.

Bipartite Patella

Bipartite patella is the most common form of multipartite conditions and occurs when there is failure of fusion of one separate center of ossification. This center is usually located in the superior lateral aspect of the patella (Fig. IV.22).

At times, in addition to independent ossification of the superior lateral pole, the area may remain unossified.

Differentiation of this entity from a fracture is based on the location of the separate fragment on the superolateral aspect of the patella, the fact that it is usually bilateral, and that the line of separation is curved with smooth dense opposing surfaces. True fracture surfaces are usually irregular, unilateral, and with no sclerotic margins.

Tripartite Patella

Tripartite patella is failure of fusion of two separate centers of ossification, giving the patella a comminuted appearance (Fig. IV.23).

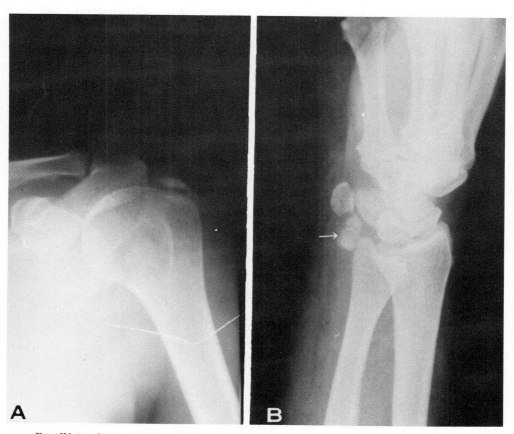

FIG. IV.21. Juxtaarticular calcification.

(A) Calcification in the supraspinatous tendon giving an appearance of an avulsion fracture of the greater tuberosity. Note, however, the amorphous appearance of the deposit and the smooth complete border of the humerus.

(B) Calcification in the tendon of the flexor carpi ulnaris giving the appearance of a dislocation of a carpal bone. Fragmentation is present suggesting that a fracture also has occurred.

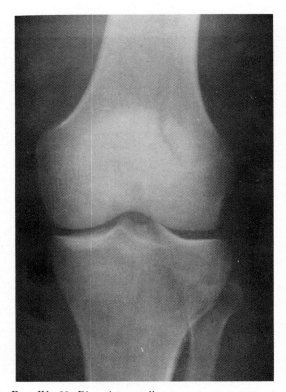

FIG. IV. 22. Bipartite patella presents as a separate
center of ossification in the superior lateral aspect of
the patella and resembles a fracture. The location and
the curved lucent line with smooth borders assist in
the   diagnosis.

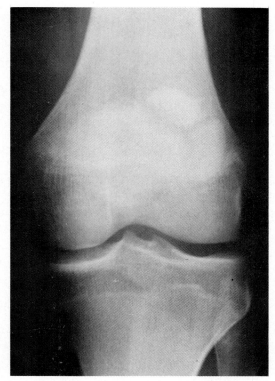

Fig. IV.23. Tripartite patella. More than one center of ossification is present, giving the patella a comminuted appearance. The location, however, is still the superior lateral aspect of the patella and comparative x-rays may assist in the diagnosis.

Again, differentiation can be made through knowledge of the fact that the anatomic variations of the patella are frequently bilateral and the opposing surfaces have smooth borders.

Differentiation of bi- and tripartite patellae and true fracture must also be made from Larsen-Johansson disease, which is osteochondritis of an infrequent accessory center of ossification at the inferior border of the patella.

Bipartite Scaphoid

Bipartite scaphoids are rare and present difficulty in differentiation from an old ununited fracture of the scaphoid. The defect is usually bilateral and this is probably the most important factor in assessing the pathology (Fig. IV.24). The history of the injury is also an important distinguishing feature. Symptoms produced by trauma to a bipartite scaphoid will most commonly subside; however, symptoms arising from an ununited scaphoid will usually be persistent. Another factor to be considered is that ununited fractures usually result in degenerative changes in the involved surfaces and adjacent bones.

Thus differentiation may be assisted by noting the bilateral nature of bipartite scaphoid with no displacement and smooth cortical edges of the adjacent surfaces, or the degenerative changes at the radiocarpal articulation and/or the presence of aseptic necrosis or cyst formation which may accompany nonunion of a fracture.

NUTRIENT FORAMINA

Penetrating the cortices of long bones are large vascular foramina for veins and arteries. These nutrient foramina enter the shaft obliquely

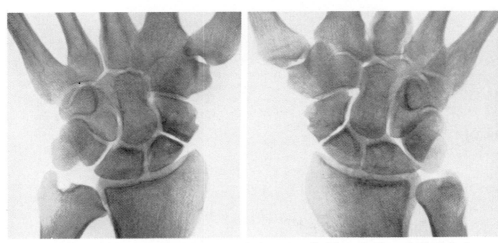

FIG. IV.24. Bipartite scaphoid. This rare lesion is usually bilateral. (From S. Brailsford: *The Radiology of Bones and Joints*, Ed. 5, p. 91, The Williams & Wilkins Co., Baltimore, 1953.)

and may be several inches in length. The obliquity of the foramina is usually directed away from the more actively growing end of the bone. At times, especially in young bones where the foramina are large, the cortical defect may be mistaken radiographically for a fracture. The diagnosis can be assisted by noting the smooth oblique appearance of the nutrient foramina as opposed to the irregular contour of a fracture, the location and the oblique direction in relation to the faster growing epiphysis (Fig. IV.25).

PSEUDOFRACTURES (UMBAUZONEN)

Pseudofractures are radiolucent zones that have been confused with, and must be differentiated from, stress fractures. They represent spontaneous nondisplaced fractures which occur in pathologic bone, especially in malacic diseases, as opposed to stress fractures which occur in normal bones. Pseudofractures are transverse lucent zones of varying widths (from less than a millimeter to more than a centimeter), usually symmetrical in distribution, and represent an area of unmineralized

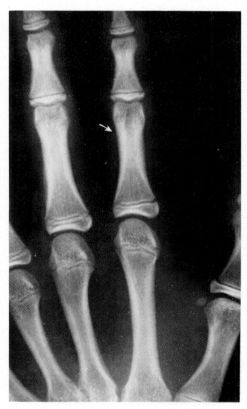

FIG. IV.25. Nutrient foramen. Note the presence of the oblique radiolucency which gives the appearance of an incomplete fracture.

osteoid (Fig. IV.26). The zones have been found most commonly in osteomalacia, Milkman's syndrome, rickets, and Paget's disease and have been termed Looser zones.

Pseudofractures differ from actual fractures in that they develop spontaneously without trauma, are bilaterally symmetrical and are usually incomplete without displacement of the fragments.

SEPARATION OF THE DISTAL TIBIOFIBULAR SYNDESMOSIS

X-rays of the ankle taken in the oblique (mortice) view may give the appearance of a separation of the distal tibiofibular syndesmosis. It should be noted that this view is designed to demonstrate the syndesmosis and thus the bones will always appear separated. An x-ray of the ankle in the anteroposterior projection will permit proper assessment (Fig. IV.27). (See "Anatomy," under "Ankle" (Section II, page 120; and Fig. II.42, page 122.

SESAMOIDS

Sesamoid bones are bones which develop in tendons and occur near a joint. By their location they serve to increase the functional efficiency

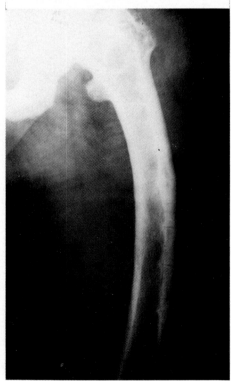

FIG. IV.26. Pseudofractures.

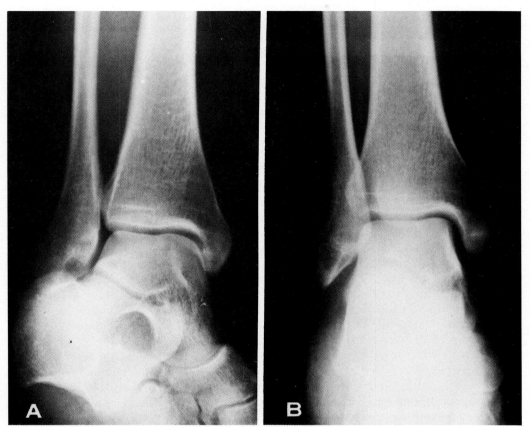

FIG. IV.27. Separation of the distal tibiofibular syndesmosis.

(A) Oblique view of the ankle mortice may give the appearance of a separation of the tibiofibular syndesmosis.

(B) On the anteroposterior projection, however, the ankle mortice is closed and there is no separation of the syndesmosis.

of the joint by improving the angle of approach of the tendon into its insertion.

Sesamoids of the Hand

The sesamoids of the hand overlie the heads of the metacarpals and the interphalangeal joints. The most common location is at the metacarpophalangeal joint of the thumb, although they are frequently found at the metacarpophalangeal joint of the small finger and the interphalangeal joint of the thumb. Occasionally, one or two sesamoids may be present at the heads of any metacarpal.

In the normal position sesamoids may be confused with avulsion fractures of the adjacent bone (Fig. IV.28). Obtaining an x-ray in several projections will assist in the diagnosis as it will demonstrate the entire outline of the sesamoid, as well as the complete outline of the adjacent bone.

Multipartite Sesamoids

The location of sesamoids in the foot is similar to the hand, that is, overlying the heads of the metatarsals.

In addition to distinguishing sesamoids from avulsion fractures, sesamoid bones themselves may be fractured. This occasionally occurs in the foot. A pitfall that may be encountered is mistaking a multipartite sesamoid (bipartite or tripartite sesamoid) for a fracture. Developmental cleavage of the sesamoids of the foot is not uncommon and usually involves the medial sesamoid. The division may be into two or more fragments. Fracture of a sesamoid is relatively uncommon and usually the result of direct trauma. Most commonly the medial sesamoid is involved (Fig. IV.29).

The differential diagnosis is difficult and perhaps to be made with reservations. A few guide lines are offered. Multipartite sesamoids are usually larger than a normal or fractured sesamoid, have smooth, more regular opposing surfaces with cortical margins, and may be bilateral. In an acute fracture, the line of fracture is sharp, irregular, assumes any shape, and may be displaced. At times, it may be necessary to see fracture healing before the diagnosis can be made.

Fabella

The fabella is a sesamoid which develops in the lateral head of the gastrocnemius muscle, approximately at the level of the knee. On lateral x-ray projection, the fabella may give the appearance of a loose body in the knee joint. Differentiation may be made by its location which is posterior to the knee joint and usually not exactly at the level of the joint line. Loose bodies on the other hand are found within the confines of the joint (Fig. IV.30).

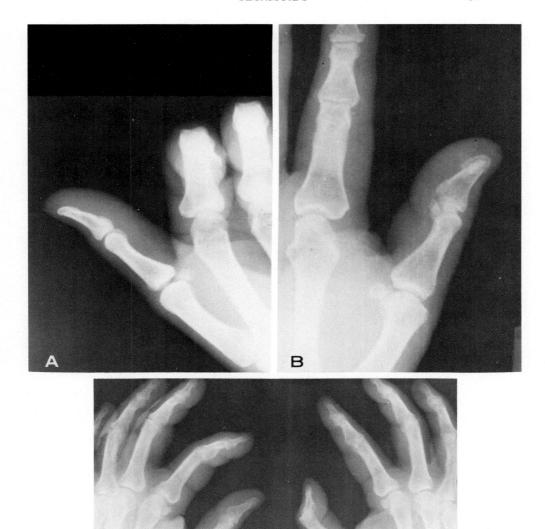

Fig. IV.28.

(A) Sesamoid adjacent to the thumb metacarpal gives the appearance of an avulsion fracture. Note that the borders are smooth however, and that the margins of the meta-carpal head are complete.

(B) Less common sesamoid than those found at the metacarpal head is adjacent to the base of the terminal phalanx of the thumb which may also resemble an avulsion fracture.

(C) Another less common sesamoid is adjacent to the head of the second metacarpal. Note the bilateral nature of this entity as well as the smooth, rounded borders which help in distinguishing this entity from a fracture.

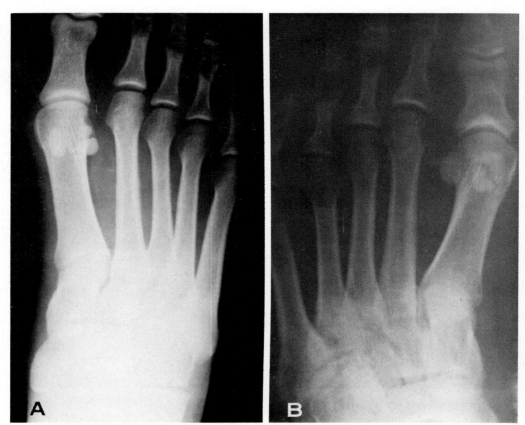

Fig. IV.29.
(A) Bipartite lateral sesamoid. Note the smooth, regular apposing surfaces.
(B) Fracture of the medial sesamoid. Note the irregular fracture line and the absence of cortical margins.

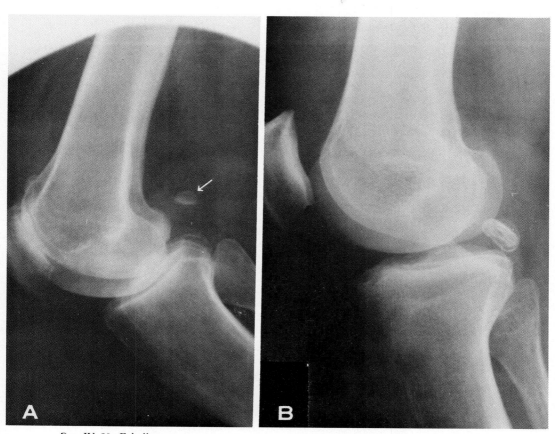

FIG. IV.30. Fabella.

(A) Location of the fabella is posterior to the knee joint and, in this case, superior to the articular surface.

(B) Loose body is located within the confines of the knee joint and at the level of the joint line.

Pisiform

The pisiform is a sesamoid which develops in the tendon of the flexor carpi ulnaris. It is located in the proximal row of carpal bones and is positioned in front of the triquetrum. This anterior position of the pisiform is normal and, at times, depending on x-ray projection, it may be misinterpreted as being dislocated (Fig. IV.31). Views in other positions will assist in making the correct diagnosis.

Ectopic calcification can occur in the tendon of the flexor carpi ulnaris and may give the impression of a dislocation or a fracture of the pisiform (see Fig. IV.21B).

SPINE

Cervical Spine

Variations in Children

X-ray examination of the cervical spine in children reveals variations which may simulate fractures or subluxations. These are related to epi-

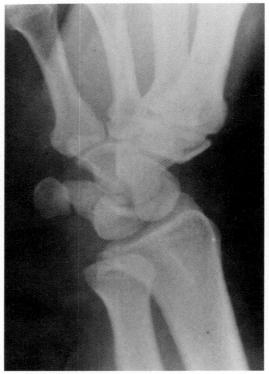

Fig. IV.31. Pisiform. The pisiform is actually positioned in front of the triquetrum and, on oblique views of the wrist, may appear as being dislocated.

physeal lines, hypermobility, and incomplete ossification. As comparative x-rays are not available in cervical spine problems, the interpretation is thus more difficult.

Hypermobility of the cervical spine in children under 8 years of age allows for additional forward movement of the axis in flexion and extension and produces an apparent subluxation of the second on the third cervical vertebra. Precise measurements from fixed points of reference will allow for the proper diagnosis.

Hypermobility also affects the relationship of the atlas and the axis (C-1 and C-2). Radiographs of the cervical spine in extension may demonstrate overriding of the anterior arch of the atlas to the top of the odontoid process, giving the appearance of a subluxation of C-1 on C-2. This also is a normal variation of the cervical spine in children (Fig. IV.32).

Epiphyseal Lines and Incomplete Ossification

In the cervical spine, there are various epiphyses which are present and may resemble fractures. For example, a cartilaginous plate is usually present at birth at the base of the odontoid and generally closes at 3 years of age. Infrequently, it may remain as a single radiolucent line which may be misinterpreted as a fracture through the base of the odontoid.

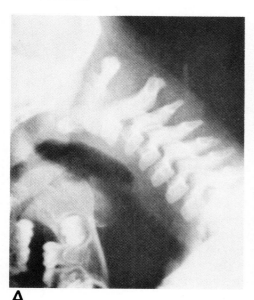 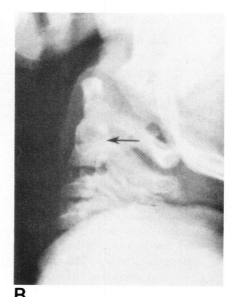

A   **B**

Fig. IV.32. Variations which may resemble subluxations in children. Flexion (A) and extension (B) x-rays of the cervical spine. (From H. S. Cattell and D. L. Filtzer: *Journal of Bone & Joint Surgery, 47A:* 1296, 1965.)

    (A) In flexion, anterior displacement of C-2 on C-3 may occur.

    (B) In extension, there is overriding of the arch of C-1 over the odontoid.

Other Lines Which Simulate Fractures of the Odontoid

The summation of shadows of adjacent structures about the odontoid may give the appearance of a fracture. These are shadows produced by teeth, air, and the arch of the axis.

Tooth Overlying the Odontoid

Frequently on the open mouth odontoid view, a central incisor may overlie the odontoid, with the inferior margin of the tooth usually appearing somewhere between the midportion and the base of the odontoid. This overlapping shadow can give the appearance of a fracture of the odontoid.

Another simulated fracture of the odontoid can result from the gap between the central incisors which may appear as a longitudinal fracture. Careful inspection will outline the appropriate shadows (Fig. IV.33).

Air Overlying the Odontoid

Air shadows from the oral pharynx and possibly the nasopharynx, if overlying the odontoid, can give the false impression of a fracture of the odontoid (Fig. IV.34). Again, careful inspection of the outline of the lucent shadow and the odontoid will allow for the proper diagnosis.

Arch of the Axis

Radiologically, on the open mouth view, the shadow of the anterior arch of the atlas can be identified crossing the odontoid. At the inferior margin of the anterior arch as it crosses the odontoid, the double density produced by the arch plus the odontoid, compared to the relative radiolucency below, can give the appearance of a fracture. Tracing the shadow of the inferior margin laterally will assist in proper evaluation (Fig. IV.35).

Ectopic Calcification

Calcification within the soft tissues adjacent to the vertebrae frequently occurs. The calcification is usually associated with osteoarthritic changes in the spine and represents calcification within the longitudinal ligaments or a degenerative intervertebral disc.

At times, the location of the calcium deposit can give the impression of an avulsion fracture. Inasmuch as the vertebrae have undergone degenerative changes, they usually have an alteration of the normal shape which thus adds to the confusion.

The diagnosis can be assisted by noting the smooth apposing borders and the absence of a nidus from which the avulsion arises (Fig. IV.36).

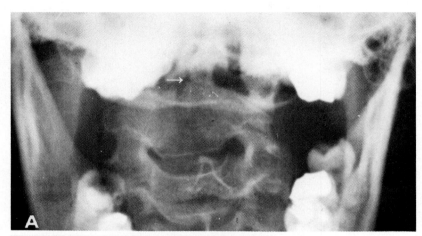

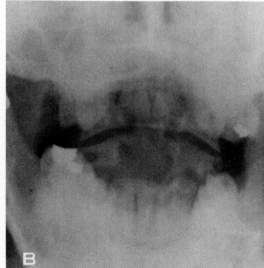

Fig. IV.33. Tooth overlying the odontoid.

(A) The distal end of the incisor when it overlies the odontoid may give the appearance of a fracture. Note carefully the outline of the tooth.

(B) Gap between central incisors may give the impression of a longitudinal fracture of the odontoid.

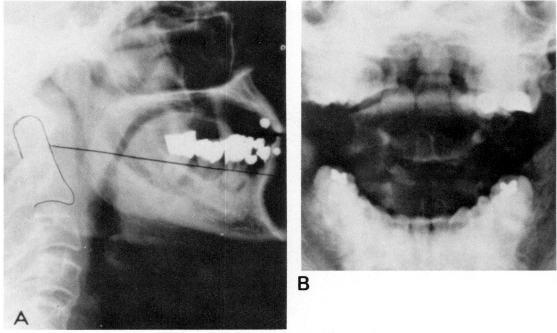

FIG. IV.34. Air overlying the odontoid. In (B) air from the oral pharanx is transecting the odontoid in its midportion simulating a fracture of the odontoid. (A) illustrates the direction of the x-ray path that produces this shadow.

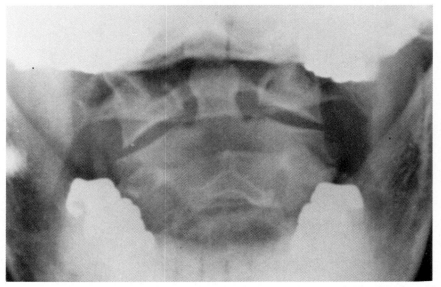

FIG. IV.35. The inferior margin of the anterior arch of the atlas as it crosses the odontoid may give the appearance of a fracture.

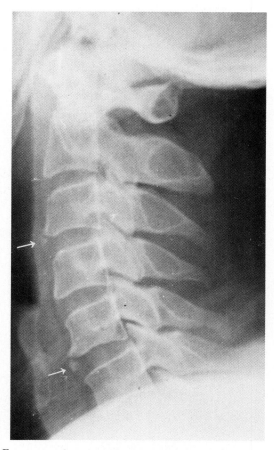

Fig. IV.36. Ossification in the anterior longitudinal ligament or intervertebral disc simulates the appearance of
an avulsion fracture. Note that adjacent to the anteroinferior margin of the third and fifth cervical vertebrae,
soft tissue ossification presents the appearance of an
avulsion fracture.

Epiphysis of the Vertebrae

See page 356.

Spondylolysis

Spondylolysis is a defect which is present in the neural arch of usually the fifth, and occasionally the fourth, lumbar vertebra, resulting in a loss of bony continuity of the pars interarticularis. The defect may also be present in any vertebrae. The pars interarticularis is a segment of bone which is located between the superior and inferior articular processes. This defect is most noticeable on the oblique x-ray of the lumbar spine. The etiology of spondylolysis is unknown; however, it probably is a developmental error. The defect may resemble a fracture; however, although this may be considered as a possible etiology, callus and fracture healing have never been demonstrated (Fig. IV.37).

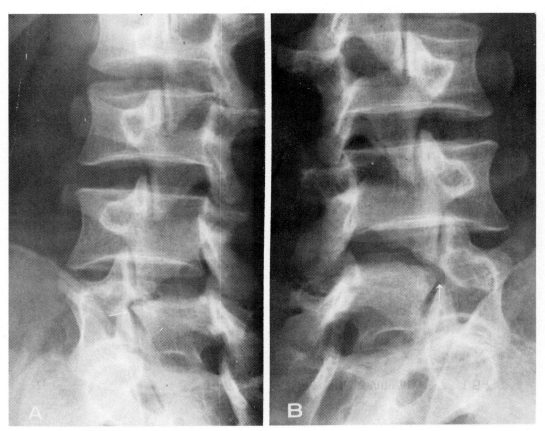

Fig. IV.37. Spondylolysis.

(A) Defect in the pars interarticularis of the fifth lumbar vertebra gives the appearance of a fracture through the pedicle.

(B) Comparative views of the other side reveals the presence of a similar defect.

Spondylolisthesis

Bilateral defects in the pars interarticularis result in loss of the stabilizing component of the posterior elements and may result in anterior displacement of the superior vertebra on the one just inferior to it. This entity, which may simulate a fracture dislocation of the spine, is called spondylolisthesis. In spondylolisthesis, the body, superior articular process, facet, and pedicle of the superior vertebrae slip forward with the inferior articular process, and spinous process remaining in their normal position. Displacement may increase gradually over a variable period of time. Differentiation from a fracture dislocation can be made by demonstrating the bilateral defect in the pars interarticularis (Fig. IV.38).

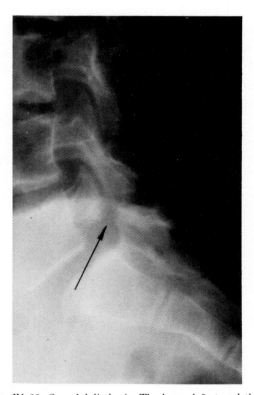

Fig. IV.38. Spondylolisthesis. The large defect and the forward displacement of the vertebrae gives the appearance of a fracture dislocation. The oblique views noted in Fig. IV. 37 demonstrate the bilateral defect in the pars interarticularis.

BIBLIOGRAPHY

Aitken, A. P.: Fractures of the Epiphyses. Clin. Orthop., *41:* 19–23, 1965.

American College of Surgeons' Committee on Trauma: *The Management of Fractures and Soft Tissue Injuries*, Ed. 2. W. B. Saunders Co., Philadelphia, 1965.

American College of Surgeons' Committee on Trauma: *An Outline of the Treatment of Fractures*, Ed. 8. W. B. Saunders Co., Philadelphia, 1965.

Anderson, H. G.: *The Medical and Surgical Aspects of Aviation*, pp. 183–194, Oxford University Press, New York, 1919.

Anson, B. J.: *Morris' Human Anatomy*, Ed. 12. McGraw-Hill Book Co., New York, 1966.

Apley, A. G.: *A System of Orthopedics and Fractures*, Ed. 3. Butterworth, Inc., Washington, D.C., 1968.

Bado, J. L.: *The Monteggia Lesion.* Translated by I. Ponseti. Charles C Thomas, Springfield, Ill., 1962.

Barr, J. S.: The Treatment of Fracture of the External Tibial Condyle (Bumper Fracture). J. A. M. A., *115:* 1683–1687, 1940.

Barton, J. R.: Views and Treatment of an Important Injury of the Wrist. The Medical Examiner, *1:* 365–368, 1838.

Barton, J. R.: Views and Treatment of an Important Injury of the Wrist. Am. J. Med. Sci., *26:* 249–253, 1839.

Bennett, E. H.: Fractures of the Metacarpal Bones. Reports of the Dublin Pathological Society. The Dublin Journal of Medical Science, *73:* 72–75, 1882.

Bennett, E. H.: On Fracture of the Metacarpal Bone of the Thumb. Br. Med. J., *2:* 12–13, 1886.

Bick, E. M.: *Source Book of Orthopaedics.* Hafner Publishing Co., New York, 1968.

Blount, W. P.: *Fractures in Children.* The Williams & Wilkins Co., Baltimore, 1962.

Boehler, L.: *The Treatment of Fractures*, Vol. III. Grune & Stratton, Inc., New York, 1958.

Bonnin, J. G.: *Injuries to the Ankle.* William Heineman Medical Books, Ltd., London, 1950.

Bonnin, J. G.: *Injuries to the Ankle.* Hafner Publishing Co., Darien, Conn., 1970.

Brailsford, S.: *The Radiology of Bones and Joints*, Ed. 5. The Williams & Wilkins Co., Baltimore, 1953.

Brostrom, L.: An Unusual Case of Osteochondritis Dissecans. Acta Orthop. Scand., *23:* 23–25, 1953.

Burns, B. H.: Diastasis of the Inferior Tibiofibular Joint. Proc. R. Soc. Med., *36:* 330–332, 1943.

Camp, J. D., and McCulloch, J. A. L.: Pseudo Fractures in Diseases Affecting the Skeletal System. Radiology, *36:* 651–663, 1941.

Cattell, H. S., and Filtzer, D. L.: Pseudosubluxation and Other Normal Variations in the Cervical Spine in Children. J. Bone Joint Surg., *47A:* 1295–1309, 1965.

Cave, E. F.: *Fractures and Other Injuries.* Year Book Medical Publishers, Inc., Chicago, 1958.

Chance, G. Q.: Note on a Type of Flexion Fracture of the Spine. Br. J. Radiol., *21:* 249–250, 1948.

Clark, J. M.: *Modern Trends in Orthopaedic Fracture Treatment.* Butterworth, Inc., Washington, D.C., 1962.

Colles, A.: On the Fracture of the Carpal Extremity of the Radius. Edinburgh Med. Surg. J., *10:* 182–186, 1814.

Colles, A.: On the Fracture of the Carpal Extremity of the Radius. Medical Classics, *4:* 1038–1042, 1940.

Coltart, W. D.: Aviator's Astragalus. J. Bone Joint Surg., *34B:* 545–566, 1952.

Conwell, H. E., and Reynolds, F. C.: *Key and Conwell's Management of Fractures, Dislocations and Sprains.* The C. V. Mosby Co., St. Louis, 1961.

Cooper, A. P.: *A Treatise on Dislocations and on Fractures of the Joints.* Longman, Hurst, Rees, Orme & Brown, London, 1822.

Cooper, A. P.: *A Treatise on Dislocation and on Fractures of the Joints*, Ed. 2, London, 1823.

Cotton, F. J.: A New Type of Ankle Fracture. J. A. M. A., *64:* 318–321, 1915.

Cotton, F. J.: *Dislocations and Joint-Fractures*, pp. 556–560. W. B. Saunders Co., Philadelphia, 1910.

Cotton, F. J.: *Dislocations and Joint-Fractures*, Ed. 2, pp. 622–626. W. B. Saunders Co., Philadelphia, 1924.

Cotton, F. J., and Berg, R.: "Fender Fracture" of the Tibia at the Knee. New Engl. J. Med., *201:* 989–995, 1929.

Crenshaw, A. H.: *Campbell's Operative Orthopedics*, Ed. 4. The C. V. Mosby Co., St. Louis, 1963.

de Lorimier, A., Moehring, H. G., and Hannan, J. R.: *Clinical Roentgenology*, Vol. 1. Charles C Thomas, Springfield, Ill., 1954.

DePalma, A.: *The Management of Fractures and Dislocations*, Ed. 2. W. B. Saunders Co., Philadelphia, 1970.

de Quervain, F.: *Spezielle chirurgische Diagnostik für Studierende und Aerzte*, F. C. W. Vogel, Leipzig, 1907.

de Quervain, F.: *Clinical Surgical Diagnosis for Students and Practitioners.* Translated from Ed. 4 by J. Snowman. William Wood & Co., New York, 1913.

Desault, P. J.: *A Treatise on Fractures, Luxations and Others Affections of the Bones*, pp. 204–209. Translated by C. Caldwell. Fry & Kammerer, Laetitia Court, Philadelphia, 1805.

Dupuytren, G.: Mémoire sur la fracture de l'extrémité inférieure du péroné, les luxations et les accidents qui en sont la suite. Ann. Med. Chir. Hop. Paris, *1:* 1–212, 1819.

Dupuytren, G.: *Clinical Lectures on Surgery Delivered at Hôtel Dieu, 1832.* Translated by H. S. Doane. De Silver & Thomas, Philadelphia, 1833.

Dupuytren, G.: *Leçons orales de clinique chirurgicale*, Vol. 1, p. 369, Ed. 2. Germer Bailliere, Paris, 1839.

Dupuytren, G.: *On the Injuries and Diseases of Bones*, p. 282. Translated by F. LeGros Clark. Printed for Sydenham Society, London, 1847.

Dupuytren, G.: Of Fractures of the Lower Extremity of the Fibula, and Luxations of the Foot. Medical Classics, *4:* 151–172, 1939.

Edwards, H. C.: The Mechanisms and Treatment of Backfire Fractures. J. Bone Joint Surg., *8:* 701–717, 1926.

Essex-Lopresti, P.: Fractures of the Radial Head with Distal Radio-Ulnar Dislocation. J. Bone Joint Surg., *33B:* 244–247, 1951.

Furlong, R.: *Clinical Surgery: Fractures and Dislocations*, p. 12. Butterworth, Inc., Washington, D. C., 1966.

Galeazzi, R.: Über ein besonders Syndrom bei Verletzungen im Bereich der Unterarmknochen. Arch. Orthop. Unfallchir., *35:* 557–562, 1935.

Gardner, E., Gray, O., and O'Rahilly, R.: *Anatomy*, Ed. 3. W. B. Saunders Co., Philadelphia, 1969.

Gosselin, L: Sur les fractures en V du tibia. Gazette des Hôpitaux Civils et Militaires, Paris, *28:* 218, 1855.

Gosselin, L.: Leçons sur les factures en vet de leurs complications. Gazette des Hôpitaux Civils et Militaires, Paris, *39:* 37, 1866.

Gosselin, L.: Recherches cliniques et expérimentales sur les fractures malléolaires. Bulletin de L'Académie de Médecine, Paris, Ser. 2, *1:* 817–826, 1872.

Gosselin, L.: Clinical Lectures on Surgery Delivered at the Hôpital of Charité. Translated by Lewis A. Stimson, p. 90, 1878.

Gosselin, L.: *Clinique Chirugicale de l'Hôpital de la Charité*, Vol. I, p. 603. J. B. Bailliére et Fils, Paris, 1879.

Grant, J. C.: *A Method of Anatomy*, Ed. 5. The Williams & Wilkins Co., Baltimore, 1952.

Grant, J. C., and Basmajian, J. V.: *Grant's Method of Anatomy*, Ed. 7. The Williams & Wilkins Co., Baltimore, 1965.

Gray, H.: *Anatomy of the Human Body*, Ed. 26. Lea & Febiger, Philadelphia, 1954.

Gunn, G.: Patella Cubiti. Br. J. Surg., *15:* 612–615, 1928.

Haliburton, R. A., Sullivan, C. R., Kelly, P. J., and Peterson, L. F.: The Extraosseous and Intraosseous Blood Supply of the Talus. J. Bone Joint Surg., *40A:* 1115–1120, 1958.

Holland, C. T.: A Radiographical Note on Injuries to the Distal Epiphyses of the Radius and Ulna. Proc. R. Soc. Med., *22*: 695–700, 1929.

Hughston, J. C.: Fractures of the Distal Radial Shaft, J. Bone Joint Surg., *39A*: 249–264, 1957.

Jefferson, G.: Fractures of the Atlas Vertebra. Br. J. Surg., *7*: 407–421, 1919–1920.

Kaplan, E. B.: *Functional and Surgical Anatomy of the Hand*, Ed. 2. J. P. Lippincott Co., Philadelphia, 1965.

Kleiger, B., and Mankin, H. J.: Fracture of the Lateral Portion of the Distal Tibial Epiphysis. J. Bone Joint Surg., *46A*: 25–32, 1964.

Kohler, A., and Zimmer, E. A.: *Borderlands of the Normal and Early Pathologic in Skeletal Roentgenology*. Grune & Stratton, Inc., New York, 1968.

Last, R. J.: *Anatomy: Regional and Applied*, Ed. 4. J. & A. Churchill, Ltd., London, 1966.

Lauge, N.: Fractures of the Ankle. Arch. Surg., *56*: 259–317, 1948.

Le Fort, L.: Note sur une variété non décrite de fracture verticale de la malléole externe par arrachement. Bulletin Général de Thérapeutique Médicale et Chirurgicale, *110*: 193–199, 1886.

Levitin, J., and Colloff, B.: *Roentgen Interpretation of Fractures and Dislocations*. Charles C Thomas, Springfield, Ill., 1956.

Lisfranc, J.: *Précis de médecine opératoire*, Vol. I. Paris, 1845.

Lisfranc, J.: *Nouvelle méthodes opératoire pour l'amputation partielle du pied dans son articulation tarsométatarsienne*. Gabon, Paris, 1815.

Lisfranc, J.: *Clinique chirurgicale de l'Hôspital de la Pitié*. Chez Bechet Jeune et Labe, Paris, 1841.

Lopez, R., and Lewis, H.: Larsen's-Johanson Disease. J. Clin. Pediatr., *7*: 697–700, 1968.

Maisonneuve, M. J. G.: Recherches sur la fracture du péroné. Archives Générales de Médecine, Ser. 3, *7*: 165–187, 433–473, 1840.

Malgaigne, J. F.: *Traité des fractures et des luxations*, Vol. I, pp. 650–656. J. B. Bailliere, Paris, 1847–1855.

Malgaigne, J. F.: *A Treatise on Fractures*, pp. 523–527. Translated by J. H. Packard, J. P. Lippincott Co., Philadelphia, 1859.

Matzen, P.-F., and Fleissner, H. K.: *Orthopedic Roentgen Atlas*. Grune & Stratton, Inc., New York, 1970.

McKellar Hall, R. D.: Clay-Shovelers Fracture. J. Bone Joint Surg., *22*: 63–75, 1940.

McLean, F. C., and Urist, M. R.: *Bone*, Ed. 3. The University of Chicago Press, Chicago, 1968.

Monteggia, G. B.: *Istituzioni Chirurgiche*, Vol. 5, pp. 129–131, Ed. 2. Maspero e Buocher, Milano, 1814.

Moore, E. M.: Three Cases Illustrating Luxation of the Ulna in Connection With Colles' Fracture. Transactions of the Medical Society of the State of New York for 1880.

Morris, J. M., and Blickenstaff, L. D.: *Fatigue Fractures—A Clinical Study*. Charles C Thomas, Springfield, Ill., 1967.

Mulfinger, G. L., and Trueta, J.: The Blood Supply of the Talus. J. Bone Joint Surg., *52B*: 160–167, 1970.

Müller, M. E., Allgöwer, M., and Willenegger, H.: *Manual of Internal Fixation*, p. 10. Springer-Verlag, New York, 1970.

Perkins, G.: *Fractures and Dislocations*. University of London, The Athlone Press, London, 1958.

Pott, P.: *The Chirugical Works of Percivall Pott*, Vol. I, pp. 433–440. Lowndes, Johnson, Robinson, Cadill, London, 1779.

Pott, P.: *The Chirugical Works of Percivall Pott*, Vol. I, pp. 433–440. Lowndes, Johnson, Robinson, Cadill, London, 1783.

Pott, P.: *Some Few General Remarks on Fractures and Dislocations*, pp. 57–64. Hawes, Clark, Collins, London, 1765.

Pott, P.: *Some Few General Remarks on Fractures and Dislocations*, pp. 57–64. Hawes, Clarke, Collins, London, 1768.

Pott, P.: *The Chirugical Works of Percivall Pott*, Vol. 2, pp. 312–317. James Williams, Hawes, Clarke, Collins, London, 1769.

Pott, P.: *The Chirugical Works of Percivall Pott*, Vol 2, pp. 312–317. James Williams, Dublin, 1778.

Pott, P.: *Some Few General Remarks on Fractures and Dislocatons.* Medical Classics, *1:* 333–337, 1936.

Provost, R. A., and Morris, J. M.: Fatigue Fracture of the Femoral Shaft. J. Bone Joint Surg., *51A:* 487–498, 1969.

Ralston, E. L.: *Handbook of Fractures.* The C. V. Mosby Co., St. Louis, 1967.

Rang, M.: *Anthology of Orthopaedics.* The Williams & Wilkins Co., Baltimore, 1966.

Rolando, S.: Fracture de la base du premier métacarpien. Presse Med., *18:* 303–304, 1910.

Salter, R. B.: *Textbook of Disorders and Injuries of the Musculoskeletal System.* The Williams & Wilkins Co., Baltimore, 1970.

Salter, R. B., and Harris, W. R.: Injuries Involving the Epiphyseal Plate. J. Bone Joint Surg., *45A:* 587–622, 1963.

Schneider, R. C., and Kahn, E. A.: The Significance of the Acute Flexion or "Tear-Drop" Fracture Dislocation of the Cervical Spine. J. Bone Joint Surg., *38A:* 985–997, 1956.

Schneider, R. C., Livingstone, K. E., Cave, A. J. E., and Hamilton, G.: "Hangman's Fracture" of the Cervical Spine. J. Neurosurg., *22:* 141–154, 1965.

Shands, A. R., and Raney, R. B.: *Handbook of Orthopaedic Surgery.* The C. V. Mosby Co., St Louis, 1967.

Shanks, S. C., and Kerley, P.: *A Textbook of X-ray Diagnosis*, Vol. IV, Ed. 3. W. B. Saunders Co., Philadelphia, 1959.

Shepherd, F. J.: A Hitherto Undescribed Fracture of the Astragalus. J. Anat. Physiol., *17:* 79–81, 1882–1883.

Smith, R. W.: *A Treatise on Fractures in the Vicinity of Joints and on Certain Forms of Accidental and Congenital Dislocation*, p. 162. Lea & Blanchard, Hodges & Smith, Philadelphia, 1847.

Smith, R. W.: *Fractures in the Vicinity of Joints and on Certain Forms of Accidental and Congenital Dislocation*, p. 162. Lea & Blanchard, Hodges & Smith, Philadelphia, 1850.

Spalteholz, W.: *Hand Atlas of Human Anatomy*, Ed. 7. J. P. Lippincott Co., Philadelphia,

Speed, K.: *Fracture Dislocations*, Ed. 2. Lea & Febiger, Philadelphia, 1928.

Speed, K.: A Discussion of Pott's Fracture with Complications Based on a Series of 208 Cases. Surg. Gynecol. Obstet., *19:* 73–82, 1914.

Stieda, A.: Barker's Arch. Klin. Chir., *85:* 815, 1908.

Taleisnik, J., and Kelly, P.: The Extraosseous and Intraosseous Blood Supply of the Scaphoid Bone. J. Bone Joint Surg., *48A:* 1125–1137, 1966.

Tillaux, P.: *Traité de chirurgie clinique*, Vol. 2, p. 842. Paris, Asselin et Houzeau, 1894.

Tillaux, P.: *Traité d'anatomie topographique*, pp. 1075–1083, Ed. 6. Paris, Asselin et Houzeau, 1890.

Tillaux, P.: *Leçons de clinique chirurgicale.* Paul Thiery, Asselin et Houzeau, Paris, 1895.

Turek, S. L.: *Orthopaedics: Principles and Their Application*, Ed. 2. J. P. Lippincott Co., Philadelphia, 1967.

Watson-Jones R.: *Fractures and Joint Injuries*, Ed. 4. The Williams & Wilkins Co., Baltimore, 1960.

Woodburne, R. T.: *Essentials of Human Anatomy.* Oxford University Press, New York, 1961.

PART I REVIEW

Fig. I.A. Open comminuted fracture of the middle and distal thirds of the first meta-carpal. Note the presence of the missel which caused the injury and the open nature of the fracture.

Fig. I.B. Complete transverse fracture of the junction of the distal and middle third of the fifth metacarpal.

Fig. I.C. Comminuted transverse fracture of the junction of the proximal and middle third of the radius and a segmental fracture of the ulna.

Fig. I.D. Spiral fracture of the distal third of the tibia and the proximal third of the fibula.

Fig. I.E. Transverse pathologic fracture through the distal third of the humerus. Note the lytic area through which the fracture passes.

Fig. I.F. Distracted, comminuted fracture midshaft of the humerus with a butterfly fragment.

Fig. I.G. Intraarticular avulsion fracture of the dorsal aspect of the base of the distal phalanx.

Fig. I.H. Comminuted intraarticular fracture of the distal radius. Note that the fracture is somewhat T-shaped.

Fig. I.I. Spiral fracture of the middle third of the tibia in good position and alignment.

Fig. I. J. Spinal fracture of the tibia with lateral angulation or medial angular displacement of the distal fragment.

Fig. I.K. Malunion comminuted intraarticular fracture of the distal femur, with lateral angulation or medial angular displacement of the distal fragment.

Fig. I.L. Nonunion of a hip fracture. Note the sclerotic margins and the occlusion of the medullary canals.

Fig. I.M. Dorsal dislocation of the interphalangeal joint of the thumb.

Fig. I.N. Fracture dislocation of the fifth metacarpocarpal joint with a comminuted fracture of the base of the fifth metacarpal and proximal and ulnar displacement.

HIP REVIEW

Fig. A. Intracapsular transcervical fracture in a child. Note the presence of the capital femoral epiphysis and the epiphysis of the greater trochanter.

Fig. B. Base of neck fracture. Note the displacement and the coxa vara position.

Fig. C. Comminuted subtrochanteric fracture.

Fig. D. Aseptic necrosis of the head of the femur. This is a subcapital fracture that had an open reduction and internal fixation with a hip nail. Note the relative increased density and irregular contour of the head of the femur. The fracture line is still visible, possibly indicating a delayed or nonunion.

KNEE REVIEW

Fig. A. Fracture dislocation of the knee. Note the depressed intraarticular fracture of the medial tibial plateau and the lateral position of the tibia.

Fig. B. Lateral dislocation of the patella on the right. Comparative view of the other knee reveals the normal position of the patella.

Fig. C. Depressed fracture of the lateral tibial plateau.

Fig. D. Y-shaped intercondylar fracture of the femur. Note the intraarticular involvement.

Fig. E. Transverse fracture of the midpatella with distraction. Note the comminution of the distal fragment.

ANKLE REVIEW

Fig. A. Minimally displaced transverse fracture of the medial malleolus.

Fig. B. Linear intraarticular fracture of the anterior aspect of the distal tibia. Only slight displacement has occurred.

Fig. C. Fracture dislocation of the ankle. Fracture of the lateral malleolus with lateral dislocation of the ankle.

Fig. D. Bimalleolar fracture with lateral subluxation of the ankle, diastasis of the inferior tibiofibular syndesmosis, and an avulsion fracture of the lateral aspect of the distal tibia. This avulsion is produced by the inferior tibiofibular ligaments.

FOOT REVIEW

Figs. A and B. Anteroposterior and lateral radiographs of a dislocation of the middle cuneiform.

Fig. C. Markedly comminuted intra- and extraarticular fracture of the os calcis. In addition, there is a transverse fracture through the neck of the talus.

Fig. D. Dislocation of the tarsometatarsal joints of the first through fifth toes with lateral displacement.

Fig. E. Transverse comminuted open fracture of the middle third of the third metatarsal. The presence of the metallic fragments indicates the open nature of the injury.

Fig. F. Comminuted intraarticular fracture of the os calcis and a comminuted fracture of the cuboid.

SPINE REVIEW

Fig. A. Fracture dislocation C-2 on C-3. There is a pedicle fracture of C-2 with forward dislocation.

Fig. B. Posterior dislocation C-4 on C-5. Note that the posterior border of the body of C-4 is not in line with the posterior border of the body of C-5.

Fig. C. Wedge compression fracture.

Fig. D. Fracture odontoid with forward subluxation C-1 on C-2.

PELVIS REVIEW

Fig. A. Comminuted fracture of the left side of the pelvis with an incomplete fracture of the superior pubic ramus, a transverse fracture of the inferior pubic ramus, and a comminuted fracture of the inferior ischial ramus.

Fig. B. Separation of the right sacroiliac joint and the pubic symphysis.

Fig. C. Comminuted fracture of the right iliac crest.

SHOULDER REVIEW

Fig A. Infraglenoid dislocation.

Fig. B. Fracture of the middle third of the clavicle on the right.

Fig. C. Anterior dislocation of the shoulder.

Fig. D. Fracture of the surgical neck of the humerus.

Fig. E. Fracture dislocation of the head of the humerus. Note that the fracture has taken place through the surgical neck.

ELBOW REVIEW

Fig. A. Incomplete, nondisplaced supracondylar fracture of the humerus.

Fig. B. Comparative view of the opposite extremity of patient in Fig. A.

Figs. C and D. Anteroposterior and lateral radiographs. Fracture dislocation of the elbow. Note that there is a posterior dislocation of the elbow with an oblique fracture of the lateral condyle.

Fig. E. Fracture of the head of the radius with inferior displacement of the fracture fragment.

FIG. F. T-shaped intercondylar fracture of the humerus.

FIG. G. Comminuted fracture of the olecranon and fracture of the coronoid processes.

WRIST AND HAND REVIEW

FIGS. A and B. Anteroposterior and lateral radiograph of transcaphoid perilunate dislocation with dorsal displacement of the carpus. Note the quadrilateral shape of the lunate on the anteroposterior projection and that the concavity is facing distally on the lateral projection. There are overlapping shadows of the capitate and proximal fragment of the navicular, and the hamate and lunate.

FIGS. C and D. Anteroposterior and lateral radiograph of perilunate dislocation with anterior displacement of the carpus.

FIG. E. Oblique fracture of the pisiform.

FIG. F. Transverse fracture through the waist of the navicular.

FIGS. G and H. Anteroposterior and lateral radiograph of anterior dislocation of the lunate.

INDEX